# SEX POSITIONS FOR COUPLES

*A guide to discover hot sex and exciting games to satisfy his/her forbidden desire. A sexy day by day guide of a modern kama sutra, tantric sex and massage secret.*

**DONNA DARE**

© **Copyright 2019 - All rights reserved.**

The content contained within this book may not be reproduced, duplicated or transmitted without direct written permission from the author or the publisher.
Under no circumstances will any blame or legal responsibility be held against the publisher, or author, for any damages, reparation, or monetary loss due to the information contained within this book. Either directly or indirectly.

**Legal Notice:**
This book is copyright protected. This book is only for personal use. You cannot amend, distribute, sell, use, quote or paraphrase any part, or the content within this book, without the consent of the author or publisher.

**Disclaimer Notice:**
Please note the information contained within this document is for educational and entertainment purposes only. All effort has been executed to present accurate, up to date, and reliable, complete information. No warranties of any kind are declared or implied. Readers acknowledge that the author is not engaging in the rendering of legal, financial, medical or professional advice. The content within this book has been derived from various sources. Please consult a licensed professional before attempting any techniques outlined in this book.
By reading this document, the reader agrees that under no circumstances is the author responsible for any losses, direct or indirect, which are incurred as a result of the use of information contained within this document, including, but not limited to, — errors, omissions, or inaccuracies.

# Table of Contents

Description ................................................................... 1
Introduction .................................................................. 5
   What Is The Kama Sutra? ........................................... 5
**Chapter 1: What Is Tantric Sex** ............................. 10
   Tips for Beginners ..................................................... 10
**Chapter 2: Prepare Mind and Body to Sex** ............. 16
   The Art of Exciting a Woman .................................... 19
   The Preliminary Games ............................................. 20
   The Orgasm .............................................................. 21
   The Multiple Orgasms ............................................... 23
   The Vaginal Pleasure ................................................ 24
   Female Ejaculation ................................................... 26
**Chapter 3: Unlocking Sexual Fantasies and Fetishes** 27
   Building Your Carnal Confidence .............................. 36
**Chapter 4: The Science behind Tantric Sex** ............ 46
**Chapter 5: Tantric Massage Techniques** ................. 62
**Chapter 6: Kinky Kama Sutra** ............................... 68
   Using the nails ......................................................... 68
   Love bites ................................................................ 70
   Woman on top ......................................................... 73
**Chapter 7: Charms, Aphrodisiacs, Artificial Membranes And Sex Toys** ........................................................ 76
**Chapter 8: 30 Kama Sutra/Tantric Positions For Best Pleasure For Him** ................................................... 100

**Chapter 9: 30 Kama Sutra/Tantric Positions For Best Pleasure For Her.................. 116**

**Chapter 10: The Benefits of Kama Sutra ............... 134**

**Chapter 11: How to Last Longer ........................... 140**

**Chapter 12: Exercises to increase male orgasmic control ...................................................................... 143**

   Kegels – strengthening the Yoni............................ 145

   Exercise for better sex ........................................... 147

   Yoga ........................................................................ 149

**Chapter 13: How to Apply Everything you've Learnt about Kama Sutra........................................... 156**

**Conclusion................................................................ 160**

# Description

Sex positions are one of the great facets that make sex wonderful. A lot of people toss between a few sex positions and never venture out farther than that for whatever reason. Some people are not comfortable trying new positions while other people live for the adventure and the challenge. Regardless of your willingness to participate, sexual positioning can stimulate and arouse areas of your body that you never knew were possible. In fact, it is well known that couples that try different sexual positions often have a lot of stronger bond and intimacy than couples that do not.

Sexual positioning allows for you to explore each other's bodies and find out what makes the other one goes over the edge. Finding out how to make your lover orgasm is arousing all in its own. One of the most wonderful things about sex is your ability to bond with one another. Introducing new sexual positions in the bedroom can bring you both closer as a couple. Communication in the bedroom is one of the most important aspects of relationships, without communication relationships will cease to exist.

This book was intended to provide you with an overview of some of the most popular sexual positions and how to implement them in your relationship. Most of these positions can be done in or outside of the bedroom and can be done with the addition of toys or nothing. A lot of these positions focus on deep penetration, which can be very beneficial to men who are trying to stimulate the woman's g-spot. One of the most difficult things for men to do is to make a woman climax during vaginal penetration, and with the use of these positions and the tips incorporated in their descriptions, having the woman orgasm is more possible than ever.

Men also need to take into account the necessity for foreplay before implementing these positions. Foreplay needs to be done for both men and women to warm them both up before sexual intercourse. Foreplay can and should include oral sex and the use of hands. Women take significantly longer to warm up than men, meaning men should get a head start in arousing the woman before they expect oral sex to begin on them (arguably). Foreplay can be one of the only ways a woman is able to climax during vaginal sex, so men need to take their time during this and put as much passion into it as possible.

When introducing sex toys during these positions, most of them allow the use of some type of toy. A common toy used in most of these positions would be the vibrating cock ring that allows for arousing vibrations for both the male and the female. The vibrating ring is especially arousing when accompanied by deep penetration, which is a feature that most of these positions offer. Another great toy to use could be a small clitoral vibrator or stimulator to help the woman climax this is especially helpful if there was not a lot of foreplay done prior to penetration.

This guide will focus on the following:

- What Is The Kama Sutra
- What is tantric sex
- Prepare mind and body to sex
- The science behind tantric sex
- Tantric massage techniques
- Charms, aphrodisiacs, artificial membranes and sex toys
- 30 kama sutra/tantric positions for best pleasure for him
- 30 kama sutra/tantric positions for best pleasure for her
- The benefits of kama sutra

- How to last longer
- Exercises to increase male orgasmic control
- How to apply everything you've learnt about kama sutra... AND MORE!!!

# Introduction

## What Is The Kama Sutra?

You might have already heard about this legendary collection of texts in pop culture. Images depicting sensual acts between consenting adults may come into mind at the mere mention of the name. In fact, several movies have already been made based on the teachings in this scripture. It might have been thrown around as a joke or two in some scenes but the term Kama Sutra has become quite synonymous to the amorous affair of making love.

Closely related to matters behind locked bedrooms, this literary piece was compiled by a sage called Vatsyayana Mallanaga for a Hindu audience.

In truth, it is impossible to pinpoint who created these writings, but the modern world is lucky that efforts have been made not just to compile them, but to translate them from ancient Sanskrit to more modern tongues.

For beginners, Hinduism is known as one of the largest religious movements in the world; third largest to be exact. Most of the people who practice Hinduism are from Nepal, India, Bali and Bangladesh.

On top of being one of the largest collections of followers in the world, it is also one of the oldest. It can be said that Hinduism stems from Vedic traditions which hail from a time wherein India had barely discovered iron and have begun utilizing it.

The Vedic tradition is known as the oldest form of worship in the Hindu world and modern Hinduism is based on its teachings. It is surprising to see that a collection of knowledge so old would still have bearings in today's society.

Interestingly, this compilation (The Kama Sutra) isn't just about elaborate measures of coital pleasure. This collection mainly talks about the regular Joe (in ancient Indian times) and how he should live his life amongst the people. It paints pictures of the modern man's life (at that time). From tending to his personal business to nights out with friends and lovers, it covers almost every aspect of a grown Indian man's life.

Not only does it talk about men. It also talks about how women should behave during those times. Think of it as a manual for day-to-day discourse and engaging members of the opposite sex.

It even contains advice on how to attract women. Needless to say, the Kama Sutra is a book about pleasure. In fact, its direct translation into English is "Treaties on Pleasure."

## History of the Kama Sutra

This collection of scriptures is only one of three ancient writings hailing back from Ancient India.

According to these scriptures, people should aspire for four goals in life; power (artha), pleasure (kama), moral obligation (dharma) and release from the cycle of reincarnation (Moksha). Each goal was inscribed in ancient texts. Unfortunately, the annals for artha and dharma have been lost in time. All that remains are the treaties on love and pleasure brought by the Kama Sutra.

Vatsyayana compiled these scriptures with his own interpretations during the $4^{th}$ century. He converted the ancient Sanskrit into a more modern Indian dialect. Many years after, British scholars went to work on creating a translated version of these documents.

The first known English publication of these writings came out in 1883. They were first published under a Sir Francis Burton who worked with Indian nationals to obtain original copies of the text to try to produce a close translation of the traditional writings.

After that, numerous other scholars came out with their own translations and versions over the following years. One popular publication entitled "The Complete Kama Sutra" came out in 1994 under the name Alain Danielou. This book originally came out in French and later translated into English. This book contained many exact texts coming from Vatsyayana and interpreted for audiences that are more modern.

**The Kama Sutra Today**

Although many things have already changed within today's millennia, plenty of people still consider the Kama Sutra as a source of relationship advice for couples. Since the book talks about courting, coitus and marriage, plenty of people think of it as classic knowledge that still applies to the modern world.

Interestingly, the sexual positions described in the manual have become a large area of interest for many modern couples looking for something to spice up their relationship. This is perhaps one of the reasons why these writings have been closely related to discussions on bedroom practices.

On another note, the challenges of modern life have also influenced the way couples communicate and express interest and affection in today's age. This also means that the problems couples face are also different. Arguments are more commonplace, cheating has become a rampant yet taboo discussion, pornography and unmentionables now plague the relationships of today.

The Kama Sutra provides a classic solution to these problems by introducing couples to a simple set of practices that can rekindle lost passions and keep both parties contented with each other; which is one of the main goals of the texts.

# Chapter 1: What Is Tantric Sex

Sting famously said mentioned that tantric sex allowed him and his wife to enjoy 7-hour sex sessions. He, later on, quipped that this time included all the begging, dinner, and a movie. The truth is that the goal of tantric sex is more about slowing things down, improving intimacy, igniting passion and improving communication as well.

If you are worried that your sex-life has become too much of routine, this is the perfect way to break the trend. This is an ancient system that has been used for thousands of years. The goal being to improve not just the sexual experience but to also improve the couple's relationship and sense of connection.

## Tips for Beginners

Make time for regular, weekly sessions – even if this means scheduling the time with your partner, make a firm commitment once a week, at a time where you can both devote a minimum of two hours to the process. The rule here – no cancelling except in a real case of emergency. Even if one or both of you is feeling tired, you still need to carry on with the session because tantric sex will help to reinvigorate the mind and body.

*Be open to experimentation* – at first, the exercises seem a little weird or even silly. You and your partner are bound to feel awkward at first but do keep at it – once the initial strangeness is out of the way, you'll start to see the benefits. It is important not to dismiss anything out of hand – if a certain exercise makes you feel uncomfortable, don't dismiss it but rather put it to one side to be tried at a later stage when you are more comfortable with the idea. Maintain a sense of playful curiousness and remember that this is meant to be fun. When you find something you both enjoy, you are winning.

*The mood is important* – this is not a wham, bam, thank you ma'am session. Spend some time getting ready for it – prepare the bedroom with clean sheets, comfortable pillows, and luxurious bed linen. Consider using an aromatherapy burner with some Ylang or Jasmine oil for a sensual aroma and set out some fresh fruit and something to drink – you will need the refreshment later. Make the bedroom a sensual sanctuary. Clear out the clutter and make the space a romantic one. Light a few candles and set up a playlist that will play throughout the whole session. Finally, get the room to a comfortable temperature.

*Have a bath* – Having a nice, warm bubble bath will help you both relax and help you to switch off from the day's worries. Have a nice glass of wine and set the mood with candles and relaxing music. Both of you can use the bath as a way to soak off the day's cares – but no sex, just yet.

*Shake to reinvigorate your body* – Shake away any remaining tension or energy blocks. Face your partner with your legs slightly bent and your feet shoulder width apart. Make a conscious effort to relax each part of your body before each of you shake for a minimum of 5 minutes. Shake your whole body and revel in the feeling of being alive afterwards. This reinvigorates you and causes tingles up and down your whole body.

*Do a meditation* – This helps to clear off any remaining mental stress and helps you to connect at a deeper level. Sit comfortably facing your partner with your eyes shut. Breathe in and out deeply. Carry on in this manner until you have forgotten the stresses of the day and are fully aware of being with your partner. If it is easier, you can also have relaxing music in the background.

Tell your partner what it is about them that you love so much – Look directly into your partner's eyes and tell them what it is that you appreciate and love about them. Be sincere and reach down deep to really let them know why you love them. This helps both of you reconnect and reminds both of you what your relationship truly means. Ask them to do the same thing and be sure to thank them when they respond.

*Eye-Gazing* – For the next 10 – 15 minutes, sit in silence and gaze into your partner's eyes. Match their breathing pattern as well. The object here is to just reconnect with one another spiritually. This is one area where couples usually have problems at first but do keep at it – you will soon get used to it.

*Getting closer* – Now it is time to practice the Yam Yum Pose – You can either do this naked or fully clothed, your choice. The man sits down with legs crossed and the woman sits on his lap, legs entwining his back. Hug each other and sit that way until your breathing synchronizes. Enjoy the closeness of this intimacy without actually involving sex.

*Tantric kissing* – Staying in the same position, with breathing synchronized, move your lip closer together and enjoy a long, sensuous kiss. Take time to really enjoy the kiss and the feelings of greater intimacy and arousal.

*Tantric massage* – you and your partner will now take turns to complete this sensual massage. The idea here is to get the skin tingling so lightly caress your partner's skin. Bring in soft flowers, sensual fabrics, feather or even ice to help ignite the senses. Start gently and gradually increase the pressure. Begin by sensuous massage of all the non-erogenous areas before you slowly move to the genitals, etc. Once the back of the body has been stimulated in this way, move onto the front. The idea behind the massage is to slowly build sexual tension. Your partner must become more and more excited and build sexual energy. They then do the same for you.

Sex – Now, if you both agree, you can move on to having slow, sensual sex. Really take your time and ensure that you both get maximum pleasure out of the session – no rushing, no worrying about who is or isn't coming. With the level of sexual tension that has built up by this stage, neither of you should have a problem coming to a climax.

After a few of these sessions, it will become easier for both of you to relax and you will find that your sexual stamina also increases.

# Chapter 2: Prepare Mind and Body to Sex

During clitoral stimulation, she keeps her eyes closed and her mouth open. Her body contracts in involuntary spasms and some women also groan. But if at some point they depart, it means they no longer enjoy the excitement and their feelings are painful or unpleasant. In most cases, only by exciting the clitoris (the main sub organ responsible for female enjoyment), women reach their climax.

Every woman wants the approach to her clitoris to be smooth – coming and going through the vulva, walking slowly and passionately through the surrounding area and, little by little, the contact getting intensified so that the desire grows as they increase the stimuli. In most cases, only by exciting this sensitive organ responsible for female enjoyment, women reach the climax. However, he can make the pleasure grow even more by enervating the nipples at the same time, caressing the contours of the anus, introducing a finger into the vagina, moistening his fingers with saliva to lubricate the most hidden folds of the vulva and the clitoris itself, as well as other points that raise the temperature and desire, as required differently by each female temperament and body.

To make sure that the intercourse gives complete pleasure to both the partners, the clitoris must continue to be excited during the penetration, being in contact and rubbing against the pelvic bone or the penis, or if the man or she caresses it.

Clitoral stimulation does not have to have as its sole objective that women are prepared for penetration or to reach orgasm. It should be taken as one of the many preliminary erotic games to enrich sensuality and increase sensitivity and confidence among lovers.

## *Excitement*

Ideally, she will openly say what gives her the most pleasure, but if she does not dare, she can guide his hand to the area she wants to be stimulated and say that she enjoys it there. The lover is not a fortune teller and female sexuality is intensely complex. No matter how much sexual experience a man has, there is always something he can learn about the art of exciting a woman.

The response to sexual stimulation begins in the mind and moves to the senses which give clear signals through the changes that are reflected in the body. The rhythm of breathing is accelerated as well as the pulse and heartbeat, and the skin turns a bit pink when blood circulation is activated. From that moment, the physiological responses are multiple: the lips take on a higher color, the pupils dilate, the nipples harden and become tense, and the skin is covered with droplets of sweat due to the increase in body temperature.

Little by little, the sense of reality is lost because the mind is completely focused on the sexual stimuli it receives. The turgor of the breasts increases and the woman feels the desire grow as the fingers rub the vulva over the clothes and the vaginal fluids begin to moisten her. The minor and major lips of the vulva swell and their hue becomes more intense. Slower to react, the clitoris hardens and grows as excitation increases. Kisses, pacifiers, and slight bites on the nipples convey pleasant sensations that grow with direct caresses in the clitoris with the fingers or tongue. Each woman has an erotic profile that marks the more or less prolonged period of stimulation necessary to be completely excited, desire penetration or reach orgasm; since there are no fixed rules, it is the lover who must discover it by himself or after being guided by her.

## The Art of Exciting a Woman

There is always something a man can learn about exciting a woman since not all of them react in the same way to stimuli and it is also not possible to awaken her desire by repeating caresses that on previous occasions have been pleasant. In each new encounter, he must learn to read the signals issued by the other body.

The excitement is not only a mechanical process of stimulation of the erogenous zones. For women, the emotional sphere and the erotic environment in which the sexual relationship occurs is very important. Although there are hidden spots especially sensitive to sensuality, which send the signals that indicate a desire to the brain, the primary erogenous zones are those that stimulate the libido and are in the genitals. When the sparks of eroticism explode, the whole body becomes receptive.

The tongue and fingertips detect the burning that invades the areas of sensitivity distinguishing, as true censors, the reactions that cause and give pleasure. From the clitoris, the enjoyment extends in concentric waves to the brain. If the caresses are distributed by all the high points, they awaken the high feminine sensibility. This is the case with the earlobe, the neck, the hollow of the armpits, and the sides of the body close to the birth of the breasts, as well as the navel since all of them are precisely the centers that respond to stimulation quickly.

The soft contact with the inside of the arms and thighs, coccyx, hips, and buttocks also unleash extremely pleasant sensations and tickles. Rubbing on the skin of the backside from the knees that descend to the legs and feet make the woman shiver and innerve by the desire that invades her.

## The Preliminary Games

She does not consider the previous games as mere preparation for the sexual act, but as the erotic moment that gradually introduces her to the enjoyment of sensations. Whether the woman already feels desire or if it is about provoking it, the erotic game of caressing, kissing, and licking the body is very suggestive and adds morbid to sexuality if one lives in fullness, without hurry and stopping in every detail and every point that can give pleasure.

She likes him to tell her how much he wants her and how he gets excited to see her and discover her while undressing her slowly and sensually. The senses come on when he rubs her breasts or pubis through the tissue and then craves to expose her bare skin to more direct and intense contact. He warns her as his breath becomes faster and begins to move with voluptuousness looking for her body. That is the moment when he slowly begins to unbutton the buttons and take off her clothes.

The act of sensually undressing women will always be exciting and not just the first time, especially if every encounter unfolds greater fantasy and the imagination is given free rein. In addition, many of them prefer to have a semi-sexual relationship or with the boom bacha on, secrets that he will know if he is attentive to the reactions. Preliminary games have no limits and cannot be planned in advance. Sometimes, they are so exciting that during previous stimulation, the woman can reach orgasm or get to the point where she ardently desires penetration.

## The Orgasm

Every moment of the excitement increases the temperature and the desire to reach the maximum sensation of pleasure. Before reaching it, the climax occurs – a peak moment that arises from the need to satisfy the body and release it from tension by exploding enjoyment.

The areolas dilate, the size of the breasts increases even more, the vaginal muscles become elastic and open to receive the penis. At the same time, the labia minora grow until the older ones overflow while the passion continues to increase. An instant before orgasm, the hardened clitoris retracts, the vagina narrows and beats hugging the phallus during intercourse, and the anal area also contracts spasm sharply. Due to the hot temperature of the skin, in some women, blush spots appear on the breasts and the back.

There are three types of female orgasm. The "resolutory" which is an intense climax that releases after the phase of desire and excitement, "Laola plateau or crest" which is less strong than the previous one but it lasts longer in successive waves of pleasure, and the "sequential or multiple" which are several successive orgasms.

She likes him to tell her how much he wants her and how he gets excited to see her, and just an instant before he discovers her, the clitoris undresses slowly and hardens. Then, it retracts sensually. Vagina narrows and beats hugging the phallus. Multi-orgasmic ability is an exclusive condition of female sexuality.

The senses come on when he rubs her breasts or pubic tissue through the fabric of her clothes.

The nipples harden and the vulva and vagina get wet. Some specialists argue that female orgasm takes longer to arrive than that of a man, but this is not always the case. Instead, everyone agrees that it is much more sensational. I will also insist on making a division between clitoral and vaginal orgasm.

The peak of sexual enjoyment is like an outbreak that produces violent uncontrolled contractions, and in some women, it is so strong that they may even lose consciousness momentarily. The more spasms are produced, the more intense and prolonged is the pleasure. From the clitoris - which is the point where orgasm is born - a sensation radiates that moves to the vulva and the vagina in a hot surge of heat that begins in the pelvic area and can spread throughout the body.

## The Multiple Orgasms

When in a short period of time a woman has a series of orgasms that occur one after another, it is said to be multi-orgasmic (an exclusive condition of female sexuality). On the other hand, males, after reaching the climax, enter a refractory period and a phase of relaxation from which they have to recover to feel excited again. However, she does not need it because of her hormonal and physiological differences. Therefore, when she has had her first orgasm, as long as it continues to excite her, others will follow.

If he is aware of the moment when she reaches the climax, the lover can enhance multiple orgasms, maintaining and increasing the stimulation without stopping. Once the first multiple orgasms have been achieved, which does not always happen from the beginning of sexual life, you can have them again. In this way, a woman's orgasmic capacity has no limits, except when her body demands rest and her energy is exhausted because pleasure has exhausted her.

## The Vaginal Pleasure

Although women have tenderness in the vagina, the center of their excitement and pleasure is located mainly in the clitoris and other erogenous points of their body. However, people have often insisted on establishing a division between clitoral and vaginal orgasm, creating a myth and generating false ideas about female sexuality that, on many occasions, can cause them to feel limited or lead them to believe that they are rare.

The truth is that the desire and passion that are aroused in the stimulated woman are transmitted to the entire area of the vulva, and the contact during penetration is pleasing because of the intimacy that it implies, although by rubbing the penis to the walls of the vagina, the woman does not have a direct sensation of pleasure, since it is a poor area in nerve endings.

The PC or pubococcygeal muscle intervenes in the increase of the sensuality of the vagina. This is found in the pelvic base and extends from the pubis to the coccyx. If the habit of contracting and relaxing it several times a day is acquired, it is strengthened and the vagina becomes more elastic. Also, by voluntarily tensing the muscles of the vaginal wall, the penis will be hugged more tightly which will cause greater pleasure in the female and male genitalia. Actually, the craving that is generated in the clitoris rises to the vagina. So, when you have a clitoral orgasm, that feeling of pleasure extends to the penetrated vagina.

## Female Ejaculation

When excited, all women produce a fluid, in greater or lesser quantity, because the blood vessels dilate and press the walls of the vagina. This liquid serves to lubricate them and facilitates penetration, creating moisture and environment conducive to enjoyment during sexual intercourse.

According to some specialists, there are women who stimulate the G-spot to eliminate a semen-like liquid through the urethra - during orgasm - which can be so abundant that it may become necessary to collect it so as not to soak the sheets. Although, it is always possible to locate this point, the vast majority of them never ejaculate.

# Chapter 3: Unlocking Sexual Fantasies and Fetishes

You probably have fantasies and fetishes you don't even know about.

They are lodged in there, in the deeper reaches of your subconscious, and simply haven't had a chance to expose them yet.

When I first started having sex, and for about a year and a half after, I had no clue I had a fantasy to dominate my partner. I didn't even know what that meant until it happened.

I didn't know that I would find it really hot to tie my partner up, and that my partner would find it really hot as well.

I didn't know that the thrill of getting caught while having sex in public would consume my thoughts for a period of time.

At this point in time, I don't have any strong role-playing fantasies. But I am completely open to them, even though my acting skills are crap.

And who knows, maybe I do have a powerful role-playing fantasy lodged in there somewhere. There's only one way to find out. I've got to try it.

## So, how do fantasies arise out of our subconscious?

I have a theory that a lot of them come from the sexual ideas we were subject to when we were growing up.

I watched a lot of porn in my pubescent days, and as you watch more and more of it, you start going deeper and deeper into the rabbit hole. That may have had an impact on my sexual psyche, and I wouldn't be surprised if it's the same for many people.

If you grew up in a sexually closed-off environment, where you were shamed for expressing your sexuality, you may have been compelled to rebel against it, becoming more open-minded and experimental in the process. So the experiences you had in your early sexual development may have had an impact on the fantasies and fetishes you have today.

If you can observe the fantasies you have today, try looking into your past and see if you can find their roots. It may help you understand why you have them, and in turn, help you understand your partner's fantasies and fetishes.

## So, if fantasies reside in our subconscious, how do we unlock them?

I believe that the key to unlock these fantasies is made out of the trust you have in one another.

As this trust builds, your mind relaxes, opening the doors to many things (sexual and non-sexual) that allow themselves to be expressed.

It may come in the form of a desire being blurted out randomly in the middle of a sexual conversation. It may come out after a few drinks and your words are flowing out more comfortably than usual. It may come out in the middle of passionate sex, when one of you screams out exactly what they want to be done do them.

As you become more comfortable having sexual conversations, that feeling of weirdness starts to go away. Discussing where you want to eat dinner and discussing a new sex toy you want to try become just as natural to talk about.

For those in casual relationships, you start to initiate these conversations more frequently with people you're attracted to, naturally filtering out the people who aren't comfortable discussing it, and naturally filtering in the people who are comfortable. This leads to increased overall sexual compatibility and openness.

These sexual conversations lead you two into the deeper reaches of your desires.

Maybe there's a fantasy you've masturbated to a few times. You begin considering asking your partner if they want to try it. You are a little bit uncomfortable because it's only something you have fantasized about. You have never considered actually making it a reality.

But you and your partner have become so much more comfortable discussing this stuff that it doesn't seem nearly as strange as it would have a while back. So you say, "What the hell, why not? Let's see where this thing takes us."

And so you discuss it, you find out that your partner has fantasized about the exact same thing. Suddenly, you both get that feeling of nervous excitement in the pit of your belly telling you that you're about to have another pivotal experience.

As you share more sexual experiences, the connection grows further. Every experience becomes your little secret that only you two have intimate knowledge about.

This permeates your connection in many ways, through inside jokes as you walk down the street, through a quick glance when someone says something related to your experience together, and through the subtleties of your sexual flow in the bedroom.

All of these things can compound upon each other, leading to spontaneous expressions of these fantasies and fetishes in the bedroom. Without any sort of premeditation, you suddenly get a desire that you've never had before.

You are naturally submissive, but at this moment in time, all you want to do is dominate them.

You have never told your partner how you want to be touched before, but you've suddenly got this unrelenting urge to be touched a certain way, so you whisper it in their ear and make it happen.

These fantasies and fetishes act like little mysteries of the subconscious. Clues pop up all around until in one instant the solution reveals itself and the mystery is solved.

It's an interesting area of sexuality to navigate. There are tons of fantasies and fetishes to choose from (well, I guess in most cases, it's not really a choice). Just go to a porn site and look at the categories. Almost every one of them is a different fantasy or fetish.

I have provided a list of these fantasies and fetishes to show you what is available, and to possibly help you realize that the ones you hold, the ones you feel the most uncomfortable about, are actually quite normal to have.

I would assume that you are certainly not the only one in the world that has this fetish. But if you are, good for you! You can be a trendsetter. There is really no reason to be ashamed of these fantasies.

If you are with a person you trust and who trusts you back, if you have solid communication going on, and if you have become more and more comfortable discussing your sex life and have shared sexual experiences, you should be in a more than ideal environment to express these desires.

Here is a list of some of the more prominent sexual fantasies and fetishes I could find. Just going through this list might unlock something for you.

- Anal sex
- Anal play
- Bondage
- BDSM (Bondage and Sadomasochism)
- Pretending you're strangers meeting each other and going home together
- Teacher and student
- Prisoner and prison guard
- Doctor and patient
- Nurse and patient
- Maid or house cleaner
- Having sex with a coworker
- Having sex with someone you have just met
- Having sex with someone older than you
- Having sex with someone younger than you (of legal age, of course)
- Having sex with multiple people at the same time
- Being completely submissive
- Being completely dominant

- Striptease
- MILFs
- Watching other people have sex
- Squirting
- Having sex on an airplane
- Orgies
- Voyeur (being watched while having sex)
- Different nationalities
- Sexy lingerie
- Gangbang
- Masturbation
- Being sexual with someone that wouldn't constitute a part of your chosen sexual orientation
- Using toys
- Filming each other
- Anilingus
- Footjobs and feet
- Dressing up in school uniforms
- Cheerleader fantasy

- Playing cop and criminal
- Hooking up with the delivery person
- Having sex in public
- Being spanked
- Thrusting into your partner's mouth
- Golden shower (peeing)
- Gagging
- Femdom (feminine domination)
- Fisting
- Deepthroating
- Talking dirty

Odds are, reading some of those may have made you feel uncomfortable. That's alright, especially if you haven't heard of them before.

Don't be judgmental, of yourself or others. It's next to impossible to control what we desire. If your partner expresses something to you that you don't feel comfortable with, react tactfully. If you don't, you could hurt them and tarnish all of the trust you have built together.

### Talking About Sexual Fantasies and Fetishes

You can sit down with your partner, write down all of the fantasies you have and would like to try, then trade papers and compare. It's usually much easier to start out communicating this way than to jump straight into a conversation about it.

But if you're comfortable enough, by all means, don't shy away from having that conversation.

## Building Your Carnal Confidence

Talking is supposed to be easy. After all, you've been doing it since you were a kid. But why on earth is dirty talking so darn hard? The truth is that even the most talkative individuals and even the most imaginative writers find playful pillow talk a bit challenging. Some words may seem erotic on print but might sound downright embarrassing when spoken out loud. Even the most sexually confident men and women will eventually come across a naughty word that would make them blush from head to toe. That's because traditionally, sex has always been about the deed.

At first, dirty talking would make you feel like you're somehow stripping your clothes off over and over again. With every word, it's like a new layer comes off and you'll wait anxiously as to how your partner will react. **Will he like it? Will she get turned off?**

So, how do you make sure that all that sexy talking won't send your lover packing?

**First, practice with yourself.**

Your vulgar vocab may initially shock you but who cares? You're the only one who'll be able to hear it anyway. Begin by masturbating. Then, start talking dirty to yourself. At this point, you don't have to have a rich vocabulary. Just use simple words. Focus on the pleasure and think out loud. Blurting out an honest sentence like: **"Oh yeah, that feels good."** is already a hundred times hotter than staying silent.

Next, imagine that you're having sex with your lover. It's what you do when you masturbate, anyway. If you're a guy, as you slip your cock into your lubed-up fist, imagine that it's her pussy. And so instead of saying: **"Oh yeah, that feels good."**, say: **"Oh yeah, your pussy feels good."**

If you're a woman, imagine his cock as you slide your fingers in and out of you. And so instead of saying:

"**Oh yeah, that feels good.**", say: "**Oh yeah, your cock feels so good.**"

Still, words like "good" are way too broad. When it comes to sexy talk, the more specific you are, the greater the impact. As you continue imagining that you're making love to your partner, describe the feelings in your head. Bring life to those sensations with adjectives.

Examples:

"Oh yeah, your pussy is so fucking **tight**!"

"Oh yeah, your cock is so fucking **thick**!"

But then again, anyone's cock can be thick. Anyone's pussy can be tight. For dirty talk to be powerful, it must hit home. Moreover, when using adjectives, you must be careful and make sure you stick to the truth as much as possible. For instance, don't describe a man's cock as "thick" when you both know that it isn't.

The next step, therefore, is to consider your partner. What's he/she like? What do you think he/she would like to hear most? What do you think he/she **needs** to hear most?

Is he's constantly worried about his size? Say something like: **"Baby, I love how your cock fits me perfectly."**

Is she self-conscious about her heavy boobs? Tell her how burying your face in them feels like heaven.

See, you're getting good at this already! As you get more comfortable and more talkative, masturbate and practice your dirty talk with a tape recorder. Listen to yourself. This way, you'll know whether you need to talk more or to talk less, to speak louder or softer, or whether you need to take the naughtiness up or down a notch.

**Form a positive attitude and an open mind.**

The source of most people's hang-ups is the idea that dirty talk somehow cheapens them, their partners, or their relationships. To become erotically eloquent, you need to get over the myth that dirty words make the act of sex unclean. One thing you need to understand is that a person's sexual persona is just one aspect of himself/herself. Who your lover is in the sack does not make up all of him/her. It is not who he/she is outside the bedroom. Your genitals are not dirty. Your partner's genitals are not dirty. By using straightforward words to refer to them (ex: cunt, penis, pussy, cock, breasts, boobs, vagina, balls, etc.), you are asserting the fact that these body parts are not to be ashamed of but instead deserve to be appreciated and therefore, mentioned.

Try this activity:

Stand naked in front of a mirror. Look at your genitals and touch them. Observe them. Determine and describe what you like most about them.

Ex:

My breasts are a nice handful. My nipples are small and pretty. I love how sensitive they are!

or

My breasts are big and generous. They're soft and bouncy and I love playing with them!

Make sure that you concentrate on the positive things. And never, ever compare yourself with the airbrushed vaginas and surgically enhanced penises in porno films and magazines. Ex: If you're conscious about how your labia minora is an outie, think about how awesome it is that your guy gets to have some flesh to nibble on during cunnilingus.

**Talk to your lover about sex. It's the healthy thing to do.**

The more comfortable you are with discussing sex with your lover, the easier it is for you to transition to dirty talking. After having sex, move close to your partner and confess to him/her how you felt. Mention the bedroom tricks and lovemaking positions that you liked the most. Tell your lover which things you want her/him to do again and again.

Ex: I went crazy when you put a vibrator on my clit while you went down on me. I can't wait for you to do it again.

Be specific. Get graphic. Sure, it was hot when your lover did it to you but hearing the act narrated through your lips will make it even hotter. Observe your lover's reaction. His/her response will help you gauge how he/she feels about smutty speech.

**Never judge.**

The bed should be a judgment-free zone. Just as you don't criticize your partner when he/she shows you his/her body, refrain from criticizing your lover when he/she bares his/her thoughts. Understand that to speak openly entails trust. To be vocal before, during, or after intercourse makes one more vulnerable. Therefore, during sexy talk, stifle the urge to laugh or to react indignantly. Don't rebuke your lover for his/her poor choice of words during sex or foreplay. Talk about it at least a few hours later.

Ex: You know when we were making love and you called me a cum dumpster? Well, that was a little too dirty for me."

**Dirty talk is not a license to be disrespectful.**

To stop dirty talk from being a tad too dirty for your tastes, create a set of rules with your partner. Talk about which words you're okay and not okay with.

Example: "I'm fine with being called a gutter whore. Just don't call me a bang hole."

Great lovemaking is all about giving and take. It's easy enough for the more talkative partner to dominate the dirty dialogue. That said, view dirty talking as an opportunity to allow the more silent person to verbalize more. It's one way to get to know your lover in a deeper sense. Don't forget to take turns and to always be on the same page when acting out roles. If one is the slave, then the other must be the master. There can't be two masters at one time. Moreover, being able to put yourself in the shoes of the listener and the talker will enable you to form a sensible perspective.

"Hey honey, let's dance the **chocolate cha cha.**"

Does this colloquial term for anal sex conjure images of feces? If it does, then you don't have to use it in your coital conversations. Feel free to make your own lust lingo that you'll feel comfortable with. Remember, the objective of dirty talk is to arouse you and not to gross you out. More than, making your own secret dirty dialect will serve to deepen the intimacy that you share with your lover.

**Once you've already gathered up the courage to talk dirty, don't make the mistake of going with the same old, same old stuff.**

Refrain from using the same phrases over and over. For God's sake, you've come so far, so don't spoil it! Strive to make yourself unpredictable. After all, dirty talking is ten times more powerful when you can catch your partner unaware. Experiment with different voices and venture out of your comfort zone. Be Casanova at one time and then a caveman the next.

When it comes to mastering steamy bedroom talk, widening your lewd lexicon is a useful weapon. For some, the penis and vagina may seem a bit too clinical. Instead of saying pussy or the commonly used cunt, experiment with other terms. (honeysuckle, juice box, Altar of Venus, etc.) Likewise, there are so many words you can use in place of cock (joystick, cum gun, fuck rod, etc.). Examine how you feel about incorporating these words into your lovemaking routine. Are they too trashy? Too clean? Too medical? Too offensive? Get a list of modern sex-related jargons and read them with your partner. Pick the ones that you think are hot. Laugh at the funny ones. Roll your eyes at the corny ones. Make it a fun thing!

How many times can you use the words "great" and "hot" and "good" before it all goes stale? Enrich your vocabulary of carnal adjectives. List down words you can use to describe your partner's vagina. Wet and slippery and warm are all fine but how about luscious, plump, succulent, lip-smacking? In the same way, hard and long are all good, but the words iron and enormous and powerful can also be used to describe a dick.

The same truth applies to when you describe your lovemaking and your climaxes. Saying **"That was amazing."** will sound wonderful the first, the second, and maybe even the third times but by the fourth time, the compliment is likely to seem more mechanical and less sincere. Use words like ground-shattering, out-of-this-earth, and spine-tingling to refer to a satisfying orgasm.

# Chapter 4: The Science behind Tantric Sex

Go back in your mind and try to remember if you have ever felt a moment of supreme sexual ecstasy? How did it make you feel? Did you feel exhilarated? Did you feel as if though you were deeply connected to the earth or your partner based on this experience of sex? Such intense sexual experiences are our greatest sources of pleasure.

At the same time, sex is considered to be something that is equally fascinating and fear-inducing in many people. We might want to indulge in sexual intimacy with all our heart but at the same time we might be avoiding it like the hounds of hell. We might wish to be touched but we might fear the vulnerability that comes along with that package. Similarly, we may want to rekindle lost passions but we might have forgotten how to set that lost spark aflame so that it would satisfy us like we want it to.

The practices of Tantra show us how to reclaim that sexual intimacy that we seem to have lost somewhere along the way. Though this might be one of the most ancient of arts, we will discover new joys of the erotic pathways and will expand those fleeting moments of sexual ecstasy into a lifetime's worth of sexual bliss.

It is truly beautiful how the old and somewhat lost art of Tantra still shines like a beacon for those who wish to reclaim control of their lives at a time when the stresses, fears and distractions of daily life threaten so many relationships daily. The age-old practice of Tantra teaches us how to open our hearts, our emotions and our sexuality as well.

## What Is Tantra?

Tantra is not a new phenomenon in Eastern cultures. However, its introduction to the West and especially the United States is relatively new. The origins of Tantra can be traced back thousands of years before the Common Era in India. It was originally introduced as a rebellion of sorts against Hinduism that posited, the way so many religions do, that sex was the route to evil and must be avoided in order to obtain enlightenment.

Tantra challenged these beliefs and emphasized that instead of taking one away from enlightenment, sexuality was actually a doorway that led straight to the divine itself. Tantra held that earthly pleasures such as eating, dancing and creative expressions were acts of great sacredness.

The word Tantra means 'to manifest, to expand and to show'. When it is held into a sexual context, this means that sex expands consciousness and weaves and brings together the polarities of the male and female body into one whole harmonious unit.

Many couples worry that they have to ascribe to the Tantric school of thought in order to apply the sexual techniques that this ancient art has to offer but their worries are needless as this is most certainly not the case. Tantric sexual practices can be applied to help you to prolong sex and to make your orgasms more intent. Just the positions and breathing techniques are enough; the rest is if you really want to get into those beliefs.

Tantra is also very good for one's health. Quite a few doctors have emphasized that sexual energy is one of the most powerful energies for creating and recreating lost health.

By practicing such techniques and indulging in tantric sex, we can tap into our own personal fountains of youth and vitality.

## How Is Tantric Sex Unique?

In the western world, sex is viewed more as a source of recreation rather than a means of transformation, The goal may be to reach orgasm and relief some feelings and cravings momentarily rather than to pleasure one's lover and especially to connect with them more fully. In short, where the Western notion of sex is greedy and only seeks personal satisfaction and fulfillment, Tantric sex teaches a person to indulge in the act as one part of a machine that needs both in order to work. Tantric sex teaches us that we are, in fact, not separate from our lover but that we are both one part of a two-piece set.

## Beginner Tantric Sex Techniques and their Relation to Scientific Intimacy

The type of lovemaking we practice in the Western world has a very distinctive start and finish, with a climax for the woman being preferred but certainly not necessary. This type of lovemaking lasting, at most, fifteen or so minutes. This is a very sad scenario for women who can take as much as 20 minutes to reach a state of arousal and thus cannot benefit from this type of lovemaking fully and has to remain unsatisfied more often than not.

Now when we compare the sex model of the western world with that of tantric sex, the sexual experience in this situation is seen as a dance that has no set beginning or end. There is no goal or finish line that one has to reach. Tantric sex is living in the moment in the truest sense of the world for the sake of a divine and exquisite union. This is why Tantric lovemaking is meditative, expressive and intimate to the highest degree. Tantric sex also deals beautifully with the problem of immediate arousal post-climax that is most common in men and makes sure that love can be extended to such a peak of sexual ecstasy that both a man and woman can experience several orgasms during a single session of sex.

**Tantra as a Cure for Premature Ejaculation**

Experts and sages of Tantra posit that tantric sex can be used to cure premature ejaculation. Doctors that practice modern medicine in the west also hold this belief. Men suffering from premature ejaculation can use tantric techniques to delay their orgasm. Advanced tantric practitioners can even have several orgasms within a single session of sex!

Though there are many advocates of Tantra, the most famous, perhaps, is the musician Sting who attributes his fulfilling sex life to Tantra. It's no surprise that even the best of the best use this ancient art that takes away insecurities and instills feelings of love, trust and mutual respect into a person and their partner. Tantra is a befitting act for people of all ages and levels of sexual experience.

The following exercises are scientifically proven to help you reconnect with your body; align it as one with the universe as well as to connect with your partner in the most intimate and profound of fashions. Remember that while practicing Tantric sex, your ultimate goal is not to reach orgasm or go through the steps of intercourse as a chore. Instead, your goal is to lose yourself into the intimacy of the act until you feel your very core beginning to open up and start overflowing with energy and love and you feel every pore of your being begin to breathe as your body finally gets satisfied in the ways it had been wanting to since long before you even realized.

Enjoy the act of giving and receiving pleasure in such ways and use a gentle touch and loving words all the while.

Remember that the best part of Tantric sex is that you do not have to meet with any set expectations. This opens the doors to communication and you can try to discover, both of you together if need be, what your partner finds most arousing.

Try and communicate with your lover for a long time, spend multiple weeks simply indulging in the Tantric Intimacy Exercises without feeling the burden to do something. Practicing such an intimacy act without the pressure to go all the way helps to relieve sexual guilt for all partners and helps to build trust and sexual desire fully.

Though there is a whole section in this book that is dedicated to sexual intimacy and tips regarding tantric sexual tips, here are some tips that have been scientifically known to trigger sexual desire and better tantric sex on the whole as well.

## Set Aside Time For Your Significant Other Each Week

No matter how much you might indulge in each other on a daily basis, plan at least one sexual rendezvous per week. Plan and specify an hour at least to be alone and together with your significant other. You will face many distractions along the way such as your children and work, etc. but you need to remember that you will not be able to benefit from Tantra if your relationship is not of the utmost priority to you.

## Work on the Atmosphere

It will not matter if you plan on indulging in your kitchen, dining room or any other room in your home. All that matters is that you treat the space as sacred as you treat your partner. Give the atmosphere importance and it will work in your favor too and you will feel relaxed and in the moment much more easily. Additionally, candies, flowers, art, music, aromatherapy candles and small food items that you both like can transform any room into a temple of sexual delight. Some people like to introduce sex toys into the play too and if done respectfully with both partners' consent, they can help to take sex to newfound heights. Even something as simple as dimming the lights and playing erotic music can help to create a welcoming environment.

## Focus on your dress

This is a very wide berth where you can play, as you like. You can dress provocatively or you can even opt for wearing nothing at all. Remember that this is mainly done to excite your partner and you can wear accessories that you might feel will excite them.

## The Exercises

If you feel that you cannot achieve a level of intimacy deep enough to let you indulge in tantric sex to the fullest, here are some intimacy exercises that can help you reach your aim of supreme ecstasy.

## Assign a Ritual

Sometimes, you might not be feeling spontaneous. For a lot of people, sex needs to be in a series of steps that are in the form of a ritual because it gives them a sense of knowing as if they are in a secure place. If that is the case with you, start your session with a regular activity that is ritualistic in nature.

This might consist of anything. Be it a simple act of feeding each other some food you both enjoy or having a nice relaxing drink when you are both not wearing clothes. A lot of couples enjoy indulging in an aromatherapy bath as it helps them to get intimate. This is a good way to get close to your partner. Water is a great relaxant and it is also, surprisingly, a drink that has some serious sexual potency.

Take care and time to wash each other with love. Be gentle or as vigorous as you see your partner is being with themselves. Giving each other a back rub is also useful and it fuses your energies. Some couples enjoy reading to each other as well. You can also try to play some music or simply put it on and dance it to it in order to get the both of you more comfortable.

Use your time together as if it were your last time together and communicate with them. Share what you love about each other and leave past grievances aside. The whole purpose of this is to allow you and your partner to make each other feel special and loved.

Don't worry if getting intimate is taking you a lot of time. The whole point is to make the lovemaking about you, rather than turning it into a mechanical way to sate your sexual desires. It is actually quite common for sexual partners to try out several different sex rituals over a period of weeks before they achieve the appropriate level of intimacy.

One piece of advice to keep in mind is that there is no way to gauge if you two are ready to have sex. At a certain point, the intimacy will have reached a level that you will just know, and within moments you will be in the throes before you know it.

## Breathing Exercises

How many times a day do you actively breathe while thinking about it? Probably not a lot of times unless you're actually having trouble doing so in the first place. However, in Tantric sex, breathing is a very important part of the sex. Applying tantric breathing techniques can also allow you to remove any distracting thoughts from your mind so that you can focus on your lover.

Here is a breathing exercise for you to try

Sit quietly and cross your legs and face your partner who should be sitting in the same position. Place your hands lightly on your legs wherever it is comfortable. Just make sure that the palms are facing up.

Meet your partner's gaze and softly inhale and exhale. Do not close your eyes, but look into your partner's eyes. It is said that the eyes are the windows to the soul, and there is a good reason that this saying holds so much weight.

Next, begin to actively breathe by thinking about your inhalations and exhalations. Match your partner's speed of breathing but try to keep it as slow as is comfortable. Remember to inhale through your nose and exhale through your mouth, and keep looking her in the eye while you synchronize your breathing patterns. Once you have breathed as one for about ten or so minutes, it is time to begin the next tantric practice.

**Erotic Touching**

Try out different types of sensual touching in order to help your partner and yourself appreciate each other. If not for sex itself taking the top spot, erotic touching would surely be the primary activity that humans engage in because it is so effective. In many ways, it is even more effective than sex itself because hands are more deft and agile!

Keep your partner going by offering encouragement. A great way to do this is to ask your partner to touch your erogenous zones. A woman would probably not know that the head of your penis is extremely sensitive and should be touched more, and you probably don't know just how much your partner would love it if you touched her clitoris. Just make sure that you ask your partner politely but affectionately (unless of course your partner would like to be commanded!) and remember to let your partner know that they are doing a good job, even if it is by moaning a little louder or being more into the sex itself.

Once the two of you have attained a suitable level of comfort, you can take a box and turn it into your little treasure trove of sexual plunder. In this box you can keep whatever you think would turn you on and would help you make the sex more interesting. Blindfolds, handcuffs, sex toys, whips, pornography, absolutely anything that you feel would be good for you and your partner during sex should go into this box. This will help both of you become more honest about your sexual preferences and will allow you to associate good sex with this box. This association will accentuate the sex because you will be immediately aroused upon seeing it.

Now you are more or less ready to start your own sexual adventures. Lose yourself into each other and you will be fine. Explore exciting and adventurous ways to fall in love and explore each other's minds and bodies. This is the last step to Tantric lovemaking.

**Basic Sex Techniques**

You have already judged the importance of preparation before tantric lovemaking. Remember that the sexual activities such as I emphasized above are especially important because their main objective is to allow the two of you to exchange the pleasure that you derive from sex and heighten your senses so that your arousal and emotional connection are that much more potent.

During these exercises, your body was establishing a personal intimacy with your partner. This will only be heightened as you both transition into a more deeply sexual connection. Sensual exercises meant to improve your emotional connection can be perceived as a form of prolonged foreplay. This helps the bodies to start anticipating the lovemaking that is about to ensure and thus hone them so that they get ready not only for sex but for Tantric sex as well.

Just keep in mind during your lovemaking that there is absolutely no way that you can do this wrong. If there is one thing that Tantra does not dictate, it is what is the correct or incorrect way to perform its techniques. All that matters is that you communicate and enjoy yourselves. Tantra is all about pleasure after all!

During your lovemaking, bear in mind that you are the ultimate controller of your sexual ecstasy. You can maintain yourself for practically as long as you want to, and the only real thing that you need to achieve is an intense climax for both yourself and your partner.

**Remain intimate**

Do not break eye contact for as long as you can maintain it without your eyes or watering or starting to laugh. This will heighten the intensity of your arousal because looking into a partner's eyes releases pleasure chemicals such as serotonin and dopamine in your brain. Remind each other that you are loved and wanted.

**Take it slow**

Taking your time is the essence of tantric sex. Try not to climax for as long as possible, don't climax until the orgasm is practically tearing you up inside, then simply let it go and lay back as the waves of pleasure crash over you!

Additionally, this will allow you to give your woman all the time she needs to achieve her own climax. Just remember, conserve your sexual energy for as long as possible by postponing ejaculation, and keep your eyes locked with hers for as long as possible.

**Regulate your breathing**

Try your best not to breathe too fast, for this might make you achieve orgasm quicker than you want to. Try to synchronize your breathing with that of your lover by inhaling when she does and exhaling at the same time as well. You can also switch by inhaling as she exhales or vice versa. This creates an incredibly seesaw of energy that would take you to unimaginable sexual heights!

**Try out new positions**

An excellent way to even the score between your masculine and her feminine energy is to give a couple of new positions a try. If you are dominant, you can try to be submissive to your lover for one session. Try to break down the sexual barriers you have created for yourself!

# Chapter 5: Tantric Massage Techniques

It's not uncommon for partners to jump straight from kissing or cuddling into having sex, but they're missing out. There is a lot more you can do with your partner than simply have intercourse, and extending foreplay can be very sexy and lead to an even hotter sexual experience overall. Erotic massage is a perfect way to get yourself and your partner aroused before sex takes place. And for couples that may not want to or be able to have traditional penetrative sex, erotic massage can serve as a way to keep their sexual connection intact and can lead to very satisfying mutual masturbation.

Erotic massage is different from ordinary massage in that the primary goal is for partners to tease and arouse each other. Some people find any kind of massage to be arousing. If this is the case for you or your partner, that's great! Try incorporating massage into your sexual activity more often to reap the benefits of this preference. If massage isn't inherently arousing for you or your partner, however, there are some ways you can take an ordinary massage and make it extraordinary and sexy.

One key of erotic massage is to make good use of *all* of the body's sensitive and sensuous spots. The genitals are an obvious erogenous zone, but there are other parts of the body with concentrated nerve endings that can be highly arousing when massaged. Fingers, toes, lips, and nipples are at the top of the list, but each person is different and your partner may have other areas on their body that they like to have massaged. Communicate with each other and do some experimentation to find out what works best for both of you. On the other hand, you or your partner may have areas of your bodies that you do not like to have touched. Make sure you communicate that information as well. Perhaps you feel uncomfortable having your stomach touched or massaged, or perhaps your partner is ticklish and prefers for you to avoid his or her feet. Tickling during an erotic massage is generally a turn-off, and prolonged tickling can actually be painful for the person being tickled. Unless you know your partner likes to be tickled, keep your massage erotic, not silly.

When you are doing an erotic massage for your partner, your hands are the most obvious tool you can use to touch and caress them. Run your hands down their body using long, luxurious strokes, make kneading motions, and touch them gently with your fingertips. Long strokes and light touches can be used almost anywhere on the body. Kneading works best for places with large muscles such as the thighs, butt, and shoulders. If your partner enjoys it, you can also use gentle, firm smacks as part of erotic massage. It's very common for people to be aroused by smacking, particularly on their butt. This erotic massage technique is also a low-pressure way to incorporate some dominance and submissiveness into your sex play if that is something that interests both you and your partner.

Hands are not the only body part you can use to perform erotic massage. If your hair is long enough, running it over your partner's body, especially their erogenous areas, can be very stimulating. You can also use your feet, particularly if your partner is aroused by feet or if you find using your feet to perform sexual acts to be pleasurable for you. Women can also use their breasts to caress their partner, while both women and men can touch their partners with their inner thighs, arms, backs, and butts. When giving your partner an erotic massage, position yourself so your groin is coming into contact with their skin. The feel of your pubic area against your partner can be very arousing for both of you. To mix things up, try incorporating sensual materials like silk, velvet, fur, feathers, or rubber into your erotic massage.

In addition to your hands, other body parts, and sensual materials, your mouth is the perfect tool for performing an erotic massage. Kissing, with or without tongue, and performing oral sex are both well-known ways to stimulate a partner, but the mouth can be used all over a partner's body to produce highly erotic effects. Concentrate not simply on the genital area, but also on the other nerve-rich areas of the body like the fingers, toes, and nipples. Massage these areas with your tongue or kiss them very erotically. You can also lick your partner all over, nibble their skin (gently, and make sure they like this first), or run your mouth softly and gently over their body.

As erotic massage moves closer to mutual masturbation or penetrative sex, you and your partner will want to concentrate more closely on the genitals. If you are massaging a man, focus on his penis. Don't just massage the tip and the shaft, but also work towards the root of the penis and the area between his legs that stretches from the base of the penis towards his anus. You can also massage his thighs and buttocks and, if he wants, incorporate some anal massage. Gently take one or both testicles in your hand or mouth and massage them. Make sure you don't bite or squeeze too hard. If you would like to continue with oral sex, this is the perfect transition point to take his penis in your mouth.

If you are massaging a woman, try starting with her on her stomach. Massage her butt and, if she likes it, run a finger between her butt cheeks and massage the area around her anus. Slide your fingers further between her legs and massage the area between her anus and her vagina. Then, turn her so she is lying on her back. Massage her groin and inner thighs, working towards her pubic area. Pull gently at the outer lips of her vulva, working towards her vagina, then stroke and tease the opening to her vagina. If you want to bring her to orgasm with your hands, move back and forth between the clitoris and the vaginal opening, stimulating them both. This is also a good transition point if you would like to perform oral sex.

Erotic massage doesn't always have to lead to penetrative sex or even oral sex. If, for medical or other reasons, you or your partner can't have sex, or if it's just been a long, busy day and you're too tired to go all the way, erotic massage is the perfect way to maintain your sexual connection. In addition, it's a good way to prolong foreplay and create higher levels of arousal, which can be particularly important for women before having penetrative sex. If you and your partner are looking to try something new in the bedroom, give erotic massage a try and figure out what works best for you!

# Chapter 6: Kinky Kama Sutra

Some of these recommendations won't be for everyone, but I'm sure they'll sound familiar to many and be welcomed by others. Even back in the times of the ancients, it seems people got up to a little strategically-placed hanky panky.

## Using the nails

Using your nails as part of your love play can be stimulating and erotic for both partners. All the same, some of us may not be accustomed to employing our fingernails in this way, so it's always good to check in with your partner on this one and ensure that everybody's on the same page and won't be unpleasantly surprised. Some of us already employ the nails as part of our sexual repertoire, but the Kama Sutra has some very explicit prescriptions for their use.

In Kama Sutra, the nails may be pressed into the flesh, used to scratch, or used to mark. While this may sound a little bit much to some of you, there is an erotic aspect to marking our partners with the nails that is worth exploring. The use of nails is always for later stage foreplay and should be reserved for the point at which you're both sensing that the next stage is at hand.

The use of nails is prescribed for several specific situations. As always, it's crucial to read the book from the standpoint of its historical setting, as modern people may view things differently. Then again, some will see in these prescriptions an application they can put to work in their own sex lives. A first coupling is one such situation. The use of the nails signifies that the encounter is one of many more to come. It's an expression of satisfaction and a physical means of bonding the partners together – almost like a brand. I'm sure most women reading this will be very familiar with the use of the nails for this purpose. It's a sexual "Kilroy was here".

Similarly, the nails can be used when one of the partners is leaving on a journey, or returning from one. The bonding aspect of the action is obvious, as well as the "branding" aspect. Finally, the nails may be employed when a couple makes up after an argument. In any of these scenarios, marking with the nails can't ever be used violently, or thoughtlessly. There is a psychological function to this aspect of lovemaking that most of us will recognize. It's intended to signify the bond between partners, but should never be overly forceful, or used without first discussing what's intended by it. It should also be pleasurable for both partners.

## Love bites

Love bites are such an important part of Kama Sutra's approach to sexuality that the book dedicates a full chapter to it. A *full* chapter! As with the use of nails, biting must be discussed prior to adding it to your sexual repertoire. It's important that both partners be on board and are willing to engage in the practice. While many of us use our teeth during the sex act, some people are uncomfortable with it and this eventuality should always be considered.

Of all the parts of the body which may be kissed, Kama Sutra counsels that almost all of them may be bitten. The exceptions include the eyes (for rather obvious reasons), the top lip and inside the mouth. Everything else is fair game!

The Kama Sutra also enumerates a variety of different love bites. All have a unique quality and role in sex play. They are as follows:

*Hidden Bite:* The skin bitten will turn red following the bite (a hickey).

*Swollen Bite:* The bite presses down the skin on both sides being bitten.

*Point Bite:* A small portion of skin is taken between only two teeth.

*Line of Points:* A small portion of skin is taken between all teeth possible, producing a line.

*The Coral and the Jewel Bite:* The lower lip is bitten by the top row of teeth (the lip is the coral the teeth, the jewel).

*Line of Jewels:* Both sets of teeth take the lower lip between them.

*Broken Cloud Bite:* With the mouth opened to varying degrees, the placement of the upper and lower rows and teeth varies. This creates an uneven effect. This type of bite is reserved for the woman's breasts, but may also be employed on the man's chest.

*Biting of a Boar:* This type of bite is also reserved for the breasts/chest and may also be employed on the shoulders. A row of bites is made. This type of bite is for lovers sharing intense passion for one another. Not to be taken lightly, needless to say!

Each of the types of bites, in Kama Sutra is to be employed on certain parts of the body, with cloud and boar being those bites I find most properly assigned. For the most part, though, these methods of love biting are to be practiced between people to whom the activity mutually appeals, never inflicted violently and always agreed upon in advance.

The Kama Sutra has some very interesting advice about the use of bites, advising that some playful aggression is desirable. For example, a point bite by a male partner should be followed by a line of points on the part of the woman. There is a one-upping suggested by the Kama Sutra that some will find very attractive in their use of biting as part of love play. The Kama Sutra also suggests that women "take their lover(s) by the hair and bend his head down, and kiss his lower lip, and then, being intoxicated with love, she should shut her eyes and bite him in various places." But it doesn't stop there.

It seems that in the world of Kama Sutra, bite marks left during the act of love are fit for viewing in public places. When lovers are out and about, showing one another their bite marks, as a way of reminding each other of their sexual encounters, is counseled. It's further counseled that when a man displays, such a bite mark to his lover that she smiles knowingly!

Further, the book suggests that the male partner should display his bites in turn. To this, the woman should give her male partner an angry look, as though annoyed.

How coy.

In terms of the Kama Sutra's philosophy of sexuality, such playfulness is part of making the love expressed in our sexuality a pursuit, which can become the glue in our intimate relationships. I can certainly see the wisdom of making our sexuality more playful and intense. By so doing, we can place our lovers at the center of our universes as our principal source of joy, amusement and mutual ecstasy.

## Woman on top

Probably one of the more surprising elements of Kama Sutra is the position of women. While there's much to dislike in terms of sexual equality (particularly the inclusion of courtesans in the picture), it's important to recognize the fact that this ancient document's places women firmly on top, sexually. Especially with respect to foreplay, the woman takes the lead and dominates sex play, with the man under her sexual control. It's the woman who is the aggressor in Kama Sutra, as the indomitable force from which men gain their power.

Power/Shakti is, in fact, the province of women. As we've seen in our reading of the story of Shiva and Parvati, Shiva could not conquer Tarakamura on his own. He needed his Shakti and that was his female consort. Through them, the creation of an ordered universe was born in the person of their child. Power became enfleshed, as Parvati was seen to be the reincarnation of a goddess, with the ability to stop the chaos of a world-dominating demon. It is from this spiritual reality that the sexual dominance of women in Kama Sutra has been established.

It's also extremely interesting that the Kama Sutra teaches that educated, intelligent women are more sexually attractive than their less intellectually-endowed sisters. A grounding in the arts and literacy are some of Kama Sutra's most powerful prescriptions to women who hope to be man magnets. This advice reveals that women of substance are also lovers to be reckoned with and highly sought after. That's quite an interesting contrast to the prevailing Western assertion concerning female sexual desirability. Women's sexual desirability is generally centered on their feigning a lesser intellectual prowess to that of the men they're with, or seek to be with. Women all over the world, under the influence of the West, are expected to model intellectual deference to men, in self-subjugation. In the world of the Kama Sutra, though, the educated, intelligent woman is the ultimate sex partner.

# Chapter 7: Charms, Aphrodisiacs, Artificial Membranes And Sex Toys

Charms; meaning certain ways in which one can lure or charm an individual into desire, were commonly used and practiced within Ancient Indian times. Modern-day spells and recipes that are focused on aphrodisiac like qualities are seen as far-fetched, though some claim they are effective. The Kama Sutra laid out a large number of recipes (or charms) that focused on the following types of spells:

"Affection for her husband

Desire of lawful progeny

Want of opportunity

Anger at being addressed by the man too familiarly

Difference in rank of life

Want of certainty on account of the man being devoted traveling

Thinking that the man may be attached to some other person

Fear of the man's not keeping his intentions secret

Thinking that the man is too devoted to his friends, and has too great a regard for them

The apprehension that he is not in earnest

Bashfulness on account of his being an illustrious man

Fear on account of his being powerful, or possessed of too impetuous passion, in the case of the deer woman

Bashfulness on account of his being too clever

The thought of having once lived with him on friendly terms only

Contempt of his want of knowledge of the world

Distrust of his low character

Disgust at his want of perception of her love for him

In the case of an elephant woman, the thought that he is a hare man, or a man of weak passion

Compassion lest anything should befall him on account of his passion

Despair at her own imperfections

Fear of discovery

Disillusion at seeing his grey hair or shabby appearance

Fear that he may be employed by her husband to test her chastity

The thought that he has too much regard for morality"

For the sake of entertainment and history, the following recipes were considered to be effective in winning over desirable individuals. Some of these recipes are seen more as experiments or placebo effect as opposed to actual reactions, but in ancient times these effects felt real. In fact, some of these recipes contain actual aphrodisiac items that can create arousal in certain individuals. Keep in mind "lingam" is the male penis and when you see Vatsyayana referring to deer women or bull-man, these are in relation to the classifications earlier on in the book. The following recipes and experiments are as follows:

"The armlet' (Valaya) should be of the same size as the lingam, and should have its outer surface made rough with globules.

'The couple' (Sanghati) is formed of two armlets

'The bracelet' (Chudaka, cudaka) is made by joining three or more armlets, until they come up to the required length of the lingam.

'The single bracelet' is formed by wrapping a single wire around the lingam, according to its dimensions.

- The Kantuka or Jalaka is a tube open at both ends, with a hole through it, outwardly rough and studded with soft globules, and made to fit the side of the yoni, and tied to the waist. When such a thing cannot be obtained, then a tube made of the wood apple, or tubular stalk of the bottle gourd, or a reed made soft with oil and extracts of plants, and tied to the waist with strings, may be made use of, as also a row of soft pieces of wood tied together.

The above are the things that can be used in connection with or in the place of the lingam.

The people of the southern countries think that true sexual pleasure cannot be obtained without perforating the lingam, and they therefore cause it to be pierced like the lobes of the ears of an infant pierced for earrings.

Now, when a young man perforates his lingam he should pierce it with a sharp instrument, and then stand in water so long as the blood continues to flow. At night, he should engage in sexual intercourse, even with vigor, so as to clean the hole. After this, he should continue to wash the hole with decoctions, and increase the size by putting into it small pieces of cane, and the wrightia antidysenterica, and thus gradually enlarging the orifice. It may also be washed with licorice mixed with honey, and the size of the hole increased by the fruit stalks of the simapatra plant. The hole should also be anointed with a small quantity of oil.

In the hole made in the lingam a man may put Apadravyas of various forms, such as the 'round', the 'round on one side', the 'wooden mortar', the 'flower', the 'armlet', the 'bone of the heron', the 'goad of the elephant', the 'collection of eight balls', the 'lock of hair', the 'place where four roads meet', and other things named according to their forms and means of using them. All these Apadravyas should be rough on the outside according to their requirements.

The ways of enlarging the lingam must be now related.

When a man wishes to enlarge his lingam, he should rub it with the bristles of certain insects that live in trees, and then, after rubbing it for ten nights with oils, he should again rub it with the bristles as before. By continuing to do this a swelling will be gradually produced in the lingam, and he should then lie on a cot, and cause his lingam to hang down through a hole in the cot. After this, he should take away all the pain from the swelling by using cool concoctions. The swelling, which is called 'Suka', and is often brought about among the people of the Dravida country, lasts for life.

If the lingam is rubbed with the following things, the plant physalis flexuosa, the shavara-kandaka plant, the jalasuka plant, the fruit of the eggplant, the butter of a she buffalo, the hastri-charma plant, and the juice of the vajrarasa plant, a swelling lasting for one month will be produced.

By rubbing it with oil boiled in the concoctions of the above things, the same effect will be produced, but lasting for six months.

The enlargement of the lingam is also effected by rubbing it or moistening it with oil boiled on a moderate fire along with the seeds of the pomegranate, and the cucumber, the juices of the valuka plant, the hastri-charma plant, and the eggplant.

In addition to the above, other means may be learned from experienced and confidential persons.

The miscellaneous experiments and recipes are as follows:

If a man mixes the powder of the milk hedge plant, and the kantaka plant with the excrement of a monkey and the powdered root of the lanjalika plant, and throws this mixture on a woman, she will not love anybody else afterward.

If a man thickens the juice of the fruits of the cassia fistula, and the eugenia jambolana by mixing them with the power of the soma plant, the vernonia anthelmintica, the eclipta prostata, and the lohopa-jihirka, and applies this composition to the yoni of a woman, and then has sexual intercourse with her, his love for her will be destroyed.

The same effect is produced if a man has connection with a woman who has bathed in the buttermilk of a she-buffalo mixed with the powders of the gopalika plant, the banu-padika plant and the yellow amaranth.

An ointment made of the flowers of the nauclea cadamba, the hog plum, and the eugenia jambolana, and used by a woman, causes her to be disliked by her husband.

Garlands made of the above flowers, when worn by the woman, produce the same effect.

An ointment made of the fruit of the asteracantha longifolia (kokilaksha) will contract the yoni of a Hastini or Elephant woman, and this contraction lasts for one night.

An ointment made by pounding the roots of the nelumbrium speciosum, and of the blue lotus, and the powder of the plant physalis flexuosa mixed with ghee and honey, will enlarge the yoni of the Mrigi or Deer woman.

An ointment made of the fruit of the emblica myrabolans soaked in the milky juice of the milk hedge plant, of the soma plant, the calotropis gigantea, and the juice of the fruit of the vernonia anthelmintica, will make the hair white.

The juice of the roots of the madayantaka plant, the yellow amaranth, the anjanika plant, the clitoria ternateea, and the shlakshnaparin plant, used as a lotion, will make the hair grow.

An ointment made by boiling the above roots in oil, and rubbed in, will make the hair black, and will also gradually restore hair that has fallen off.

If lac is saturated seven times in the sweat of the testicle of a white horse, and applied to a red lip, the lip will become white.

The color of the lips can be regained by means of the madayantika and other plants mentioned above.

A woman who hears a man playing on a reed pipe which has been dressed with the juices of the bahupadika plant, the tabernamontana coronaria, the costus speciosus or arabicus, the pinus deodora, the euphorbia antiquorum, the vajra and the kantaka plant, becomes his slave.

If food be mixed with the fruit of the thorn apple (dathura) it causes intoxication.

If water be mixed with oil and the ashes of any kind of grass except the kusha grass, it becomes the colour of milk.

If yellow myrabolans, the hog plum, the shrawana plant, and the priyangu plant be all pounded together, and applied to iron pots, these pots become red.

If a lamp, trimmed with oil extracted from the shrawana and priyangu plants, its wick being made of cloth and the slough of the skins of snakes, is lighted, and long pieces of wood placed near it, those pieces of wood will resemble so many snakes.

Drinking the milk of a white cow who has a white calf at her foot is auspicious, produces fame, and preserves life.

The blessings of venerable Brahmans, well propitiated, have the same effect.

There are also some verses in conclusion:

'Thus have I written in a few words the "Science of love", after reading the texts of ancient authors, and following the ways of enjoyment mentioned in them.'

'He who is acquainted with the true principles of this science pays regard to Dharma, Artha, Kama, and to his own experiences, as well as to the teachings of others, and does not act simply on the dictates of his own desire. As for the errors in the science of love which I have mentioned in this work, on my own authority as an author, I have, immediately after mentioning them, carefully censured and prohibited them.'

'An act is never looked upon with indulgence for the simple reason that it is authorized by the science, because it ought to be remembered that it is the intention of the science, that the rules which it contains should only be acted upon in particular cases. After reading and considering the works of Babhravya and other ancient authors, and thinking over the meaning of the rules given by them, the Kama Sutra was composed, according to the precepts of Holy Writ, for the benefit of the world, by Vatsyayana, while leading the life of a religious student, and wholly engaged in the contemplation of the Deity.'

'This work is not intended to be used merely as an instrument for satisfying our desires. A person, acquainted with the true principles of this science, and who preserves his Dharma, Artha, and Kama, and has regard for the practices of the people, is sure to obtain the mastery over his senses. 'In short, an intelligent and prudent person, attending to Dharma and Artha, and attending to Kama also, without becoming the slave of his passions, obtains success in everything that he may undertake.'

An ointment made of the tabernamontana coronaria, the costus speciosus or arabicus, and the flacourtia cataphracta, can be used as an unguent of adornment.

If a fine powder is made of the above plants, and applied to the wick of a lamp, which is made to burn with the oil of blue vitrol, the black pigment or lamp black produced therefrom, when applied to the eyelashes, has the effect of making a person look lovely.

The oil of the hogweed, the echites putescens, the sarina plant, the yellow amaranth, and the leaf of the nymphae, if applied to the body, has the same effect. A black pigment from the same plants produces a similar effect.

By eating the powder of the nelumbrium speciosum, the blue lotus, and the mesna roxburghii, with ghee and honey, a man becomes lovely in the eyes of others.

The above things, together with the tabernamontana coronaria, and the xanthochymus pictorius, if used as an ointment, produce the same results.

If the bone of a peacock or of a hyena is covered with gold, and tied on the right hand, it makes a man lovely in the eyes of other people.

In the same way, if a bead, made of the seed of the jujube, or of the conch shell, be enchanted by the incantations mentioned in the Atharvana Veda, or by the incantations of those well skilled in the science of magic, and tied on the hand, it produces the same result as described above.

When a female attendant arrives at the age of puberty, her master should keep her secluded, and when men ardently desire her on account of her seclusion, and on account of the difficulty of approaching her, he should then bestow her hand on such a person as may endow her with wealth and happiness. This is a means of increasing the loveliness of a person in the eyes of others.

In the same way, when the daughter of a courtesan arrives at the age of puberty, the mother should get together a lot of young men of the same age, disposition, and knowledge as her daughter, and tell them that she would give her in marriage to the person who would give her presents of a particular kind.

After this, the daughter should be kept in seclusion as far as possible, and the mother should give her in marriage to the man who may be ready to give her the presents agreed upon. If the mother is unable to get so much out of the man, she should show some of her own things as having been given to the daughter by the bridegroom.

Or the mother may allow her daughter to be married to the man privately, as if she was ignorant of the whole affair, and then pretending that it has come to her knowledge, she may give her consent to the union.

The daughter, too, should make herself attractive to the sons of wealthy citizens, unknown to her mother, and make them attached to her, and for this purpose should meet them at the time of learning to sing, and in places where music is played, and at the houses of other people, and then request her mother, through a female friend, or servant, to be allowed to unite herself to the man who is most agreeable to her.

When the daughter of a courtesan is thus given to a man, the ties of marriage should be observed for one year, and after that, she may do what she likes. But even after the end of the year, when otherwise engaged, if she should be now and then invited by her first husband to come and see him, she should put aside her present gain, and go to him for the night.

Such is the mode of temporary marriage among courtesans, and of increasing their loveliness, and their value in the eyes of others. What has been said about them should also be understood to apply to the daughters of dancing women, whose mothers should give them only to such persons as are likely to become useful to them in various ways. Thus end the ways of making oneself lovely in the eyes of others.

If a man, after anointing his lingam with a mixture of the powders of the white thorn apple, the long pepper and, the black pepper, and honey, engages in sexual union with a woman, he makes her subject to his will.

The application of a mixture of the leaf of the plant vatodbhranta, of the flowers thrown on a human corpse when carried out to be burnt, and the powder of the bones of the peacock, and of the jiwanjiva bird produces the same effect.

The remains of a kite who has died a natural death, ground into powder, and mixed with cowach and honey, has also the same effect.

Anointing oneself with an ointment made of the plant emblica myrabolans has the power of subjecting women to one's will.

If a man cuts into small pieces the sprouts of the vajnasunhi plant, and dips them into a mixture of red arsenic and sulphur, and then dries them seven times, and applies this powder mixed with honey to his lingam, he can subjugate a woman to his will directly that he has had sexual union with her, or if, by burning these very sprouts at night and looking at the smoke, he sees a golden moon behind, he will then be successful with any woman; or if he throws some of the powder of these same sprouts mixed with the excrement of a monkey upon a maiden, she will not be given in marriage to anybody else.

If pieces of the arris root are dressed with the oil of the mango, and placed for six months in a hole made in the trunk of the sisu tree, and are then taken out and made up into an ointment, and applied to the lingam, this is said to serve as the means of subjugating women.

If the bone of a camel is dipped into the juice of the plant eclipta prostata, and then burnt, and the black pigment produced from its ashes is placed in a box also made of the bone of a camel, and applied together with antimony to the eye lashes with a pencil also made of the bone of a camel, then that pigment is said to be very pure, and wholesome for the eyes, and serves as a means of subjugating others to the person who uses it. The same effect can be produced by black pigment made of the bones of hawks, vultures, and peacocks.

Thus end the ways of subjugating others to one's own will.

Now the means of increasing sexual vigour are as follows

A man obtains sexual vigour by drinking milk mixed with sugar, the root of the uchchata plant, the piper chaba, and liquorice.

Drinking milk, mixed with sugar, and having the testicle of a ram or a goat boiled in it, is also productive of vigour.

The drinking of the juice of the hedysarum gangeticum, the kuili, and the kshirika plant mixed with milk, produces the same effect.

The seed of the long pepper along with the seeds of the sanseviera roxburghiana, and the hedysarum gangeticum plant, all pounded together, and mixed with milk, is productive of a similar result.

According to ancient authors, if a man pounds the seeds or roots of the trapa bispinosa, the kasurika, the tuscan jasmine, and liquorice, together with the kshirakapoli (a kind of onion), and puts the powder into milk mixed with sugar and ghee, and having boiled the whole mixture on a moderate fire, drinks the paste so formed, he will be able to enjoy innumerable women.

In the same way, if a man mixes rice with the eggs of the sparrow, and having boiled this in milk, adds to it ghee and honey, and drinks as much of it as necessary, this will produce the same effect.

If a man takes the outer covering of sesamum seeds, and soaks them with the eggs of sparrows, and then, having boiled them in milk, mixed with sugar and ghee, along with the fruits of the trapa bispinosa and the kasurika plant, and adding to it the flour of wheat and beans, and then drinks this composition, he is said to be able to enjoy many women.

If ghee, honey, sugar and licorice in equal quantities, the juice of the fennel plant, and milk are mixed together, this nectar-like composition is said to be holy, and provocative of sexual vigor, a preservative of life, and sweet to the taste.

The drinking of a paste composed of the asparagus racemosus, the shvadaushtra plant, the guduchi plant, the long pepper, and licorice, boiled in milk, honey, and ghee, in the spring, is said to have the same effect as the above.

Boiling the asparagus racemosus, and the shvadaushtra plant, along with the pounded fruits of the premna spinose in water, and drinking the same, is said to act in the same way.

Drinking boiled ghee, or clarified butter, in the morning during the spring season, is said to be beneficial to health and strength and agreeable to the taste.

If the powder of the seed of the shvadaushtra plant and the flower of barley are mixed together in equal parts, and a portion of it, i.e. two palas in weight, is eaten every morning on getting up, it has the same effect as the preceding recipe."

As you can probably see, most of these recipes are outrageous and foolish, though some state that the effectiveness of them cannot be compared. Modern-day medicine doesn't offer much of an option for men looking to enlarge the size of their penis, so recipes such as these give hope to men who aren't as well-endowed as others and who are ashamed.

Now, switching back over to modern times, there are a lot of modern-day aphrodisiacs and toys that can be used to spice up the sex life in the bedroom outside of outrageous and difficult concoctions. Some proven aphrodisiac foods are:

Oysters – who would have thought? They contain high amounts of zinc that help with fertility along with a wide range of amino acids that are said to aid in the arousal of the individual.

Chili peppers are another unexpected aphrodisiac, they are said to be the food of love because of their bright, red color. This food also mimics how one feels when aroused by speeding up the heart rate and causing you to perspire; both of which happen when one is aroused.

Avocado is another aphrodisiac due to the high amounts of Vitamin E. It is unclear how or when the arousal occurs with this food but the rich yet mild taste makes it easily morphed to taste like nearly anything it's added to.

We all know about the sexual effects of chocolate. Many have said that consuming chocolate actually gives people the feeling of being in love. Chocolate releases dopamine into the body, creating a euphoric sensation upon consumption. This is often why chocolate is used in the bedroom during foreplay as a syrup or a chocolate powder.

Bananas are said to be aphrodisiacs as well due to the triggering of testosterone production in males and the elevation of energy due to the high amounts of potassium and Vitamin B. Not only is this food healthy for you, it can also be consumed a variety of different ways.

Another fun ingredient to use in the bedroom that is also arousing is whipped cream. We aren't talking about the cheaper, zero-calorie whipped cream either. You want the rich, real whipped cream that you either make yourself or purchase from your local grocer.

Pine nuts and pumpkin seeds are surprising aphrodisiacs as well. Both high in vitamins and minerals that aid in sexual functioning such as zinc and magnesium, these nuts are easily incorporated into a variety of different recipes due to their milk flavors.

Among other aphrodisiac foods are honey, arugula, watermelon, coffee, figs, strawberries, artichokes, chai tea, cherries, pomegranate, red wine, salmon, walnuts, and vanilla.

Moving on to sex toys; today there exists more sex toys and variety than ever before. With the emergence of extreme, lifestyle sex toys in the form of robotic-like women that not only move in sexual motions but also speak and have flesh like skin covering them. Some men keep these robots in their home as replacements to women, though these are extreme cases. More regular sex toys involve a variety of different items like the "cock ring".

This ring can be purchased as a one-time use ring or multiple use. Some of the rings are simply made to squeeze the male penis to keep more blood in the shaft which is especially helpful for men who have difficulty maintaining an erection. The ring helps to keep blood in the shaft and can also vibrate if the vibrating model is chosen. When the ring vibrates, the women can feel it when the male is inside of her adding extra sensation to the act of intercourse. Aside from aiding in the sustainment of an erection, these rings also give the man more sensation because of the heightened blood flow to his penis.

Dildos and vibrators can be used by both men and women during sexual intercourse. Dildos don't normally vibrate but they simulate the shape and feel of a real-life penis. Vibrators can be small or shaped like a male penis while also having the option to vibrate or rotate. Some of these toys have grooves, notches and lumps on them for added sensations. Men can insert these items into women either vaginally or anally during foreplay or intercourse and women can insert these into the male anally during intercourse if he desires.

These toys are great when the male isn't in the mood for intercourse because he can still help the woman climax by inserting the dildo or vibrator inside of her.

Another male toy is the prostate plug; it's a butt plug that is inserted into the male anally and intended to touch or rub against his prostate during intercourse or masturbation which can be highly pleasurable. Some of these prostate plugs even vibrate, creating a nearly unbearable euphoria. Butt plugs can also be used by women to help loosen the anus for penetration or longer ones can be inserted to touch the g-spot through the colon during intercourse. One thing to be careful with is making sure that what you are using is actually intended to be inserted anally.

Devices and toys that are created to be inserted anally come with a safety type guard that prevents them from being sucked up into your anus. Because your rectum is an exit rather than an entrance, it acts as a vacuum when anything foreign is inserted (which is why you are able to hold in your feces if you aren't near a bathroom). Muscle memory will assume that the foreign object is feces and will suck it back up into the rectum, causing a dangerous and potentially lethal situation if damage or tearing occurs. Only insert anally if it says it can be inserted anally.

More items can be used such as costumes and different types of bondage items like whips, handcuffs, gag balls, collars, edibles, etc. Those types of items are generally practiced by experienced couples who enjoy bondage and not by people who are unfamiliar or put off by bondage type attire.

# Chapter 8: 30 Kama Sutra/Tantric Positions For Best Pleasure For Him

Men don't usually suffer from not being able to achieve orgasm, but there are positions that are a lot more pleasurable for them than others. Erectile dysfunction can be a psychological problem, so men suffering from this ailment should see a doctor to figure out how to close off their minds while they're enjoying a romp between the sheets. Other than that, have fun with these positions that are just as pleasurable for men as they are for women!

**Cowgirl**

Also known as girl on top and discussed in the previous chapter, cowgirl is where the woman straddles the man while he's lying down and she's facing him. Why is it pleasurable for the man? The woman is doing all the work! Most of the physical movements are going to be made by the woman, but if you feel bad, you can always join in by grabbing her hips and thrusting up. This position also allows for the most penetration for a man, so it's the best stimulation for him.

If the woman is self-conscious about her body and you cannot convince her to try this position, try reverse cowgirl. It has all the same benefits for both partners, and the woman gets to show off her sexy back.

## Around the Bend

Men love to experience deep thrusting as this is the most primal urge they have. Unfortunately, most traditional positions prevent men from going all the way in, which can leave a little something to be desired when it comes to sex for men. This position, however, alleviates all those concerns! Just position your female partner over a piece of furniture and have her spread her legs a little. Then thrust into her gently at first, and slowly build up to going into the hilt.

If the woman feels that there isn't enough intimacy, slowly lower yourself over her so that your front is touching her back. Reach around and hold her around the middle as you thrust into her to keep her steady.

## Inverted Rear

The man should lie down on his back and have his partner lie on top of him while she is facing the ceiling. He can grab onto her thighs and spread her legs until she's in a reverse straddle. In her position, she will not be able to do much when it comes to thrusting or moving, so the man has to do all the work. Once she's in the right position, the man can thrust as deeply as he wants, for as long as he wants.

One problem with this position is that if the sex is wild, it's difficult for the woman to stay balanced. The man can keep a firm grip on her thighs as he's thrusting to ensure she doesn't fall off.

**Full Mast**

For this position, the woman is going to need to be limber. While your partner is lying on her back, place her legs at a ninety-degree angle to her body. Kneel in front of her and place her legs on your chest. Then thrust deeply and slowly until the woman is ready for more.

Sometimes, when men get a little overzealous about this position, they tend to raise the woman's back off the mattress at an odd angle. So be sure to give her extra support if this happens.

**Lotus**

Just like with the cowgirl position, this position has the woman doing almost all the work. The man sits cross-legged on the bed or on the floor and pulls her into his lap. The idea is to have the woman straddle the man with her legs around his waist, and then position herself up and down until both partners have achieved orgasm. If the woman is having trouble moving up and down, a rocking motion is just as efficient.

As a tip, have the man lean against a wall during this position. This supports his back and gives her something to hold onto, which makes it easier for her to move about.

**Doggie-Style**

Mentioned in the previous chapter, doggie style is definitely the staple of a man's repertoire for dirty, naughty sex. Men get a really great view of the woman from behind and they have control over how deep and how fast they thrust during this position. It's the straight to orgasm move for a man.

Women tend to complain that they feel they're just an object during this position, and there is a lack of intimacy. That's because men tend to go through the motions and don't really get into any other kind of contact. So, men reach forward and give a gentle tug on your lady's hair or try some mild spanking.

**His Pleasure Matters!**

Gentleman and ladies, a man's pleasure matters just as much as a woman's. Yes, there are positions that are more pleasurable for a woman that are not as great for a man, even if he achieves orgasm in the end. The act is not completely about the end result, but also about feeling connected and having a great time as you're getting to that orgasm. So women should be just as conscious of their man's pleasure as their man is of theirs.

Men should not be afraid to ask their partner to try something new or to focus a little on themselves at times. After all, just like women, men are responsible for their orgasms, too.

## Packed position

The packed position is when the female extends her thighs and rests them each one on top of the other. The male can take her thighs in his arms and enter her while on his knees, kneeling.

## Lotus-like position

The lotus-like position is a highly sensual position, allowing both partners to be face to face with one another, embracing and kissing one another. The male will sit down, crossing his legs widely. The woman will sit in his lap, facing him and wrapping her legs around his back. While sitting down, she will lower herself onto his penis. This is also a deep penetration position and can be painful for men with larger penises. The woman can move up and down or back and forth while also getting clitoral stimulation from rubbing against the male's pubic region due to the positioning.

## Turning position

Requiring a relative amount of physical strength from the male, this position has been referred to in modern times, quite accurately I might add, as "the helicopter". The man will insert himself inside the woman as if performing missionary position. From there, he will remain inside the woman while turning in a circle. Think of the woman as the body of the helicopter and the male as the top propeller for the helicopter. The penis is what is keeping this helicopter connected. This position appears to be intended more for show and experimentation than actual sexual pleasure.

## Congress of a cow

The congress of a cow is actually an oral sex-driven position that is a spin-off of the sixty-nine position (69). In this position, the male will lay on his side and the woman will lay on her side as well, facing him but at the opposite end. Her face should be facing his penis and his face should be facing her vagina. From here, the male will wrap his arms around the woman's pelvis and proceed to perform oral pleasure on the woman while the female performs oral pleasure on the male.

**The visitor**

The visitor is a position that can be done standing up if you both are the same height, or it can also be done with the woman's bottom resting on the edge of the table if the male is significantly taller than she is. In this position, the male will step closer to the female, embracing her as if to hug her and placing his hands on her lower back. She will move one of her thighs in between his legs with her other leg still located on the outside of his legs. She will insert him inside of her and wrap her arms around his neck, gently moving up and down. This position works well if the male has a longer penis and if both individuals are the same height.

**The toad**

The toad, although not a very appealing name, is a deep penetrating sexual position that also allows for a great deal of intimacy. This position is initiated with the female laying on her back as if to perform the missionary position. Once on her back, the male will come at her, inserting himself inside her and stretching his legs out straight behind him. She will then pull her legs up higher and move her pelvis up and down while he is inside her. He can wrap his arms around her neck and she can reciprocate or grab his bottom. This sexual position is incredibly intimate and can also be relatively painful if the male has a longer penis so proceed gently at first.

**Bandoleer**

The bandoleer is similar to other sexual positions we have discussed, only a few different placements of the feet and hands make this position even more erotic. The female will lay on her back and pull her feet up to her chest. The male will kneel and insert himself inside her. She will place her feet on his pectoral muscles and he will cross his arms, placing each elbow on one of her knees and lifting her pelvis slightly. You can also place a pillow underneath her head for added comfort. The male will then thrust in and out slowly or in quick, short thrusts – whichever is preferred.

**The slide**

The slide is another sexual position that requires both individuals to lay on top of one another, laying out straight. This time though, the female is going to be on the top instead of the male. While the male is laying on his back, the female is going to lay on top of him in the same manner, wrapping her arms around his neck and lifting her pelvis up and down while he is inside her. Again, this is one of those positions that is best performed by people of similar length and with a meal who has a longer penis.

**The rider**

The rider is essentially the reverse cowgirl. The man will lay flat on his back and the woman will straddle him, facing towards his feet. She will place her hands on his ankles and use her knees to push herself up and down. The male can also help when she gets tired. This gives the guy a great view while also giving the woman some control on penetration and speed.

**The kneel**

The kneel is an interesting position that is also a bit difficult to describe. To start, both lovers will be on their knees. The male will sit back on his calves, almost like kneeling. The woman will move in closer, straddling one of his kneeled legs and inserting him inside of her. He can wrap his arms around her back while she wraps her arms around his neck. Either he can thrust up and down or she can, it really depends on who is being the dominant force in the position.

## The curled angel

The curled angel is a sweet sexual position that can be easily transitioned to after spooning. The position requires the male and female to both be lying on the sides, facing the same direction. The man will be behind the woman and the woman will pull her legs up to her chest, almost like the fetal position. The man will pull his legs up as well but will fold his legs with hers (his knees will be touching the back of her knees) and he will insert himself inside of her. He can lean up on his arm to get a better view of the woman and her breasts or he can lay down next to her and wrap his arm around her, embracing her.

## The grip

One of the few positions formed with the male in the doggy style position, this position requires the male to bend over on his hands and knees over the woman. She will then thrust her pelvis into the air with her arms at her sides, thrusting him inside of her. From this position, you don't have to exert a lot of force but you are still able to get deep penetration and a great view. Either the male or female can thrust, rock back and forth or work together simultaneously.

## Afternoon delight

Perfect for an afternoon quickie, this position requires the male to lay on his side and the woman to lay on her back, sitting on the male's penis. She will throw her legs over his hips while he thrusts in and out. This position is easily done on the bed and is another easily transition from the spooning position.

## The eagle

A very popular position for many reasons. The eagle position has the female on her back with her legs spread open while the male inserts himself inside her from the front. He will grab her thighs and continue to thrust into her while her legs are spread open, giving him an amazing view of penetration, her clitoris and her breasts and face during intercourse. She also has the freedom to stimulate her clitoris if necessary to achieve climax.

## The sphinx

An interesting rendition of the highly popular, doggy style position, the sphinx involved the woman laying on her stomach, sitting up on her elbows. She will then pull one leg up to her side and leave another leg stretched. The male will then put his weight on his hands, leaning over her with his legs stretched behind him, inserting himself inside her. He will then move up and down, thrusting gently. She can also help take some of the strain off of him but bouncing back onto him instead of having him do all the work.

## The column

This position involved both parties standing up, the male behind the female. The male will then insert himself inside her from behind, wrapping his hands around her waist and placing them on her pubic region. She can place her hands over his or on a surface in front of her. The position is great for a couple who wants to have a quickie.

## The clasp

This position requires either a relatively strong man or an incredibly light woman (or a combination of the two). The woman will wrap her legs around the man's waist, putting him inside of her. He will then hold her up, placing his arms on her bottom and lifting her up and down on his penis. If the weight is too much, this position can be modified by having her sit on a flat surface such as a tabletop or a counter – though the position will go by a different name if that's the case.

## The seated ball

Another intimate sexual position, the seated ball requires the male to sit on his bottom, legs stretched out in front. The woman will then sit down in the man's lap, facing the same way. She will pull her legs closer to her chest, keeping them on the outside of his legs. She will then lean slightly forward and grab his ankles while he leans forward onto her back. This is an easy position for the woman to take control and guide the male into her on her terms, not his. This position requires a bit of strength and flexibility on the woman's part but don't let that keep you away from trying a modified version.

## The perch

Using a chair as a perch, the man will sit on the chair (or stool) and have the woman sit down onto him, letting him inside her. She will be facing the same way he is, both of them placing their feet on the floor. He can wrap his arms around her waist and stimulate her clitoris or she can stimulate her clitoris while he holds her breasts. Though not a lot of visual stimulation, this position allows for a lot of touch on the male's part, giving him free rein over her body.

**The plough**

This position requires a bit of strength on both parties, along with a lower surface such as a bed. In the position, the woman will lay on the edge of the bed on her stomach with her legs straight out behind her, opened slightly for the male to walk in between. As the male walks in between, he will hold her legs up, taking some of the pressure off of her. He will lift her pelvis up so that he can put himself inside her while she balances on the bed on her arms or elbows. While the man is standing, holding her hips with her pelvis in the air, he will then begin thrusting (or ploughing) into her. The term comes from the way in which the man is holding the woman, almost as if he is plowing a field or using a push mower. This requires arm and abdominal strength and stamina from the woman as well as arm strength from the male.

**The fan**

This position is another spin-off of the commonly known and incredibly loved doggy-style position. The woman will bend forward onto a stool, table, counter, or other hard surface that is lower than she is. From this position, she will arch her back, lifting her bottom higher in the air and giving the man a much better angle for entering her. He can place his hands on her bottom or wrap them around to stimulate her clitoris (even better if this is done during anal sex). This is called the fan because the man can thrust in a circular motion, similar to a fan.

**The bridge**
This sounds difficult because it is difficult. This can only be performed by a man who is capable of maintaining the weight of their female lover on their abdomen while also performing a backbend. This position requires the male the put himself in a backbend and have the woman climb onto him, placing her hands on his pectoral muscles and moving back and forth on his penis. For an added workout, the male could attempt to thrust in and out as well, though that is highly unlikely to be pleasurable. This position will be even more difficult if the female is short and unable to reach the ground while on top of the male, meaning the male will have to hold the entire weight of the woman while maintaining his back bend. Do not attempt this if you are unsure of your strength.

**The crouching tiger**
This sexual position is another form of reverse cowgirl. The male will lay on his back on the edge of the bed, letting his feet touch the floor. From here, the woman

will climb onto his lap on reverse cowgirl position, pulling her feet up beside her and using them to move up and down as opposed to being on her knees. From this position she can stimulate either her own clitoris or fondle her lover's testicles. When her legs get tired, the male can take over and thrust while the woman lifts her pelvis slightly above his pelvis, giving him room to thrust. This position doesn't require must strength on the males side but it does require a bit of leg strength from the woman's side.

# Chapter 9: 30 Kama Sutra/Tantric Positions For Best Pleasure For Her

Everyone wants to be able to bend their bodies into different positions and angles for sex, but if women want to reach orgasm, they and their partners need to keep it simple. Wild, crazy, I never knew I could bend that way sex is excellent for keeping things interesting and on fire, but if you want to break an orgasm record, you're going to need the basics only.

When you attempt to twist into those positions and figure out new ways to have sex, your mind is concentrating on that rather than on the sex itself. The simplest positions are usually the best positions for orgasm, and with some modifications, you can make them even more orgasm-inducing than they already are.

With these sexual positions, you're going to need a little more balance and flexibility to get it right without causing damage to you or your sex partner. The precarious position certainly adds to the excitement and provides a whole new angle to the sex. However, it's best to attempt this when you've tried the beginner positions and had no problem performing them to perfection.

So here are some of the best positions for women when they want to achieve orgasm.

**Reverse Chair Sex**

Think Chair Sex but with the girl facing backward, her hands holding onto the back of the chair as the male enters from behind. It has all the benefits of deep penetration but with the added excitement of falling off the chair. From this position, the guy can play with the girl's clitoris as the female holds tights to the chair. However, there may be no option to play with female hot spots since the male needs to help maintain the balance with each thrust. Most of the movement must be centered along the pelvis since a full-body thrust may topple the girl over.

**Climbing the Tree**

Requiring balance from both the male and the female, Climbing the Tree is basically standing sex without the benefit of a wall. According to the Kama Sutra, this position provides a different kind of orgasm due to the sexual pleasure along the spine. In this situation, the male is the Tree that the female climbs with the penis acting as a branch that prevents her from falling. One of the girl's legs is hitched around the hips of the male while the other maintains balance. In this position, the male is free to play with the K-Spot, stimulate the breasts with his mouth or engage in all manners of kissing and licking.

**Almost 69**

This position starts off like the Reverse Cowgirl but instead of the female staying upright, she continues to lie down to her stomach so that her face faces the feet of the male. In this position, both the girl and the boy control the movement as the female hooks her arms around the male's calves for leverage. The guy can hold onto the girl's hips to enforce more control and guide the rhythm and depth. For guys who love female ass, this is an ideal position – not to mention the fact that it lets them see the in and out movement of the penis. The only spot the guy can hit during the Almost 69 is the K-Spot although the girl can make an effort to brush her clitoris against the male with the movement.

**The Bend**

Not exactly a difficult sex position, The Bend at least requires the female to be a little bit flexible. The male will also need to exert a bit more power as he bends the female's legs backward as he enters her from the front as you can see from the picture. This offers deep penetration and really keeps the vagina tight around the penis. Unfortunately, it's a little tough to hit the clitoris in this position but the female can play with her nipples in this position.

## So Close

Have the male sit down on the bed, his thighs opened wide as the female straddles him, making them face to face. The girl then lies down on the space between the thighs and bends her knees for leverage and control. The male also helps with the depth and rhythm of the sex by holding on to her hips and waist. With a little bending forward, the guy can play with her nipples using his mouth.

## The Lotus

Most sexual positions require the female to be flexible but in the lotus, the male must be able to open his legs wide in a lotus position. If you've seen the position of the legs during yoga, this is exactly how it looks. The female then straddles the male, her breasts meeting his chest and getting as close as possible to effect penetration. The female wraps her thighs around the male as he controls the movement of the thrust. Women can also choose to brace their feet on the floor to help with the movement. In this position, guys can easily suck on the breasts, play with the K-Spot or perhaps do lots of smooching as they try to capture a steady rhythm to capture an orgasm. It can be tough for the guy but the open leg approach offers a different kind of pleasure for the lady. In this position, the head of the penis also gets lots of attention.

**Pray It Out**

The male kneels on the bed as the female straddles him and assumes the same kneeling position. Both are capable of controlling the thrusts but most of the works is done by the guy. In this position, couples can have one powerful kiss as the guy uses one hand to handle the K-Spot. The breasts are crushed on the guy's chest or if he's a breast man, he can also choose to suck on them as he penetrates her back and forth.

**Doggy on Pillow**

Think doggy position but more comfortable for the female as she gets down on her knees while the male enters from behind. The difference here is that the female lays down her upper body on a bunch of pillows so that she doesn't have to use her hands for leverage. In this position, the male can play with her nape, stimulating this erogenous zone until both reach orgasm. It takes a little bit of balance and control on the part of both male and female to get this position right. Also, it's not the kind of position that allows you to smack your partner with powerful thrusts so guys will need to be a little gentler in this position.

**Flipped Almost**

Think Flipped 69 but this time, with the guy taking the top space and the female occupying the bottom position. The guy does most of the work but unfortunately, this doesn't leave much room for additional stimulation. Girls, however, can massage the buttocks of their partner and if they happen to be sensitive in this area, then it will definitely be a plus. If you can, try playing with the balls as they become exposed in this position. A lot of girls, however, aren't exactly fond of the view this position provides.

*Pivot*

The pivot takes into account the changing of the position from one to another. Generally, it starts off in a Doggy Position with the female keeping her legs spread open. While remaining embedded in the vagina, the female slowly uprights her upper body and the male adjusts his own posture, slowly bending backward and bracing his hands on the bed to accommodate their combined weight. In this position, the knees remain bent and as much as possible; the penis remains lodged in the vagina. The female's feet are now firmly planted on the bed, her hands stretched backward and holding onto the male arms for balance as they continue their sexual thrusting. In this position, the female is free to play with her breasts or clitoris. If capable, the guy can try bracing with just one hand and use the other for pleasure giving to his partner.

**Stool Sex**

Stool Sex works pretty much the same way as chair sex except the female's feet are planted firmly on the ground, her upper body bent downwards and holding onto a stool as the male enters her from behind. The lower height of the stool means the hips are tilted upwards, giving the guy one amazing angle to play with. Thrusting too much is not a good idea in this position since a stool isn't exactly a stable place for the girl to hold on to. On the plus side, this offers the guy a chance to hit that elusive G-Spot, especially if you happen to be long and thick. Couples who are into anal sex may also find this a favorite.

## Wheelbarrow

You've probably heard of the wheelbarrow which is actually a classic when it comes to difficult sex. It requires strength, mainly on the part of the female because she'll be supporting herself largely on her arms as the male controls the thrusting movement of the sex. In the wheelbarrow, the female goes down on all fours as the male's stands on the back. He then lifts the legs of the female and enters her from behind in a standing position.

There are several variants to the wheelbarrow. The male can either be kneeling or standing up. Depending on his position, the female can stretch out both hands to hold herself upwards or simply use pillows under her chest area to lift herself up. The typical wheelbarrow position consists of the legs opened wide and stretched straight upwards as the male holds onto the hips to maintain position. However, women have the option of keeping their knees tucked in so that the legs are bent. For others, one leg may be stretched out while the other is bent and tucked forward. These changes in leg position helps control the depth, pace, and control of the male so women are perfectly free to grab whatever position they want.

## Dolphin

Dubbed as the dolphin, this sex position starts off looking easy but can actually be tough over time. The male is basically kneeling on the bed, his thighs and upper body held straight upwards. The female is lying on her back as her hips are tilted upwards to straddle the male thighs and effect penetration. As a result, the female is basically arching her back while keeping her shoulders flat on the bedroom. The male handles the depth and penetration by holding onto her buttocks for balance.

## Wheelbarrow

The wheelbarrow functions much like the reverse of the dolphin and is equally complicated. It starts off with the female going on all fours at the edge of the bed. The then positions from behind and grabs her legs to put them around his thighs. The tough part comes when the male basically coaxes the girl to move backward so that the lower half of her body is now off the bed and completely supported by the guy. Using her hands, the female plants them on the bed as the male straddles her from behind, her legs and hips dangling off the edge. In this position, the guy again gets most of the work and doesn't leave any room for additional stimulation.

**Riding the Horse**

Definitely one of the most difficult sexual positions today, it's a little confusing why anyone would try doing this particular sex act – unless the couple is really into excitement. It works much like the Bridge which is illustrated below but is more precarious on the part of the girl. It starts off with the male supporting himself on his feet and hand in such a way that the penis is thrusting out upwards. The girl starts by straddling him from this position and then deftly lowers herself in such a way that one leg is between the thighs of the guy while the other is planted firmly on his upper body. The girl then leans backward and supports herself with one hand stretched out to the floor. In Riding the Horse, most of the job is done by the female since the male is mainly occupied with keeping himself upright. Undoubtedly, this position requires strength and stamina on both the girl and boy. On the plus side, it makes for an excellent core and arm exercise.

*Bridge*

The bridge is terribly complicated and requires flexibility and strength from the guy. The male basically arranges himself into an arch; his body fully bending backward until the only things supporting him is his hands and feet. The female then straddles him from this position and uses her leg for balance and leverage. The hands need to be used for additional balance so it's unlikely that the female would be able to pleasure herself using her hands. Still, it's an interesting position that should be tried out at least once.

Most other positions are essentially a variation of one of the positions mentioned in this chapter as well as the preceding two. Hence, couples are advised to play and experiment with the different positions available to them, bearing in mind mutual pleasure in the act. Remember though that complicated sexual positions can cause injury for some people so unless you have the strength and flexibility to make them work, it's best to stick to the basics and postpone the experiment until you're both capable of the deed.

**Curled princess**
She curls up, on her side, with her slender knees drawn up to her breast level, as her man gets inside from her behind. This can be comfortable for pregnant women too. This is a unique side posture for couples to make love in a romantic manner.

**Different Variants of doggy postures**
Women enjoy some variants of doggy postures, because they want their men to be sexually thrilled.

In normal doggy posture, the woman gets down on her palms and soft knees, as her man enters her flowery vagina from her behind.

In *Leap frogging posture*, the woman rests on forearms and elbows along with feet or knees. She rests her head on a pillow. This posture allows variation in angle of penis insertion, providing stimulation to women as well as men.

Woman can *stand and lean against the wall* or pillar; man holds her from shoulders and enters from the rear powerfully. She can be more active during his thrusts.

If the woman prefers to lie on the bed, man can lie down on top, supported on knees and ankles, or he can kneel in between her legs, depending on the angle of entry that is stimulating for each of them. He can look for her Gspot stimulation in experimenting with the angle of the penetration. Lubricating the entry point for vaginal as well as anal penetration becomes critical.

Rear entry in sitting posture, can be adopted on the side of bed or on chair, man is supported by his palms on his backside.

Woman mounts, facing his feet, knees folded and thighs pressing his thighs, her hand on his knees to make powerful thrusts.

**rock the knee posture**

Man lies on his back, with legs stretched in front. He bends his legs with strong knees pulled upwards. His naughty woman lands on him, with her warm yoni (vagina) ready to suck his erect penis, facing his feet. She holds his knees for support as she rocks her hips up and down. As he is aroused strongly to see her enchanting bare buttocks, he fondles her breasts with all his strength to make her scream.

Then she takes up face to face posture, holding his knees with elbows, leaning slightly forward.

**Widely opened position**

In order to perform this position, the woman should place a pillow under her head for comfort. Lying on her back, the man will kneel down in front of her and she will arch her back up, leaving her arms at her sides and placing her hands on his thighs. He will then insert himself inside her, gently moving up and down on. If his legs become tired, she can move her pelvis up and down. He can place his hands on either side of her back.

## Yawning position

The yawning position requires the lady to lie on her back. Her legs are extended straight in front of her, resting the back of her legs on the front of the kneeling man's legs. While he is kneeling in front of her, he will insert himself inside her and will put his hands out. She will lace her fingers with his and using the leverage of her legs, he will lean forward to penetrate deeper inside of her.

## Indrani

For this position, the woman lies on her back with her legs pulled up towards her chest. The man kneels in front of her, leaning his weight onto the back of her thighs. He will then place his hands on the outside of her knees. Placing a pillow underneath her head will help her stay comfortable. This position is intimate and with the right flexibility, couples can lock lips while performing this position.

## Clasping position

The clasping position is most easily done with the male on the top. This position can be tricky to do and requires the right anatomy to have it done correctly; i.e., average to longer penises work best in this position. The woman will lay on her back, legs straight out in front of her, flat on the ground. The man will lay the exact same way on top of the woman, inserting himself inside her. This position is not meant for deep penetration but it's a wonderful position for intimacy as far as kissing and stroking one another. The roles can also be reversed where the man is on the bottom and the woman is on top.

## Mares position

The mare's position requires the woman to be on top, straddling the male. While straddling, the man is on his back, thrusting his pelvis upward into the woman. He can hold her hips or her arms, whichever he prefers. This position allows for deep penetration.

## Rising position

The rising position is done by the woman laying on her back. She arches her back up in a wide "v" like position. This position is similar to previous positions except instead of the male thrusting into the woman, the woman thrusts her pelvis upward. She hangs onto the man's arms while he leans over her, almost as if in missionary position.

## Pressed position

The pressed position is another position that allows for deep penetration. The woman lays on her back and pulls her knees up to her chest. The kneels in front of her and grabs her knees, she places her hands on his hips. This position gives the woman the freedom to stimulate her clitoris or touch the male in different areas such as is chest, nipples, and abdomen.

## Half pressed position

The half-pressed position is a bit difficult to explain but incredibly pleasurable. This position requires the female to lay on her back, her right leg pulled up towards her chest. The male will kneel in front of her, placing his left leg outside of her right leg and extending his right leg back behind him. The woman will take her left leg and rest it over the back of the male's right leg. She can place her hands on his torso or on her clitoris for added stimulation. From here, the male will thrust into the woman.

## Splitting of a bamboo

For the splitting of the bamboo sex position, this requires the female to lay on her side, one leg stretched upward and the other straight out flat. The man will kneel in between her legs; one on either side of her pelvis. From here, she will rest her leg that is in the air on her lover's chest while he thrusts himself into her. This gives both parties a significant amount of contact making this position more intimate than others. The male can also use his hand to stimulate her clitoris or touch her breasts.

## Fixing of a nail

The fixing of a nail sex position requires a bit more flexibility than others. Described best by Yvonne K. Fulbright, PhD, MSEd, a nationally known sex therapist and author of several books on sexuality, states that "Once she is lying on her back, her lover takes one leg up and moves her into a split, stretching her leg up vertically. As he kneels around her pelvis, he rests her foot against his forehead and begins to penetrate. She then alternates legs, placing her foot against his forehead and placing the first leg flat, and then repeating. This changes the angle of each thrust, with her lover's chest against the back of her thigh moving her up and down."

## Crabs position

The crabs position is an interesting spin on the cowgirl position. This position requires the male to lay on his back while the female sits facing the male, placing a foot on either side of the male's head. He will grab onto her thighs with his hands and she can grab his shins with her hands. This position is also great for deep penetration and gives the male a great view of the woman's body and of the penetration. The couple can rock back and forth or the woman can hold herself up while the male thrusts himself upward, into her.

# Chapter 10: The Benefits of Kama Sutra

Kama Sutra is a very wonderful text that teaches us a lot about sex. As lovers, it is important that you take the teachings of Kama Sutra seriously so that you would be able to create a more stable relationship. As you already know, the Kama Sutra goes far deeper than talking about sex. Although the book talks about sex positions, the book also makes emphasis on ways of having a satisfying sex life. Following the Kama Sutra teachings, you stand a chance to become more educated about male and female. Here is some truth about the Kama Sutra you probably didn't know.

*1. Kama Sutra values empowering women*

Despite all what our modern-day society keeps preaching about women and sexuality, Kama Sutra has a different view on this subject matter. Kama Sutra suggests that a woman needs to study the different forms of sex before she gets married. When a woman understands the different forms of sex, she would be a better mate and would be more desirable by her man. So, the Kama Sutra encouraging women and empowering them is one of the biggest benefits you stand to gain from the book.

**2. Kama Sutra makes a clear classification of a man's penis**

Also, the Kama Sutra made mention of the size of a man's penis and that it matters when choosing a mate. There are three types of man penis by Kama Sutra – the bull, horse, and hare. Kama Sutra also made mention of different sizes of woman's vagina, and that a perfect match of the vagina size and penis sizes would result in a good sexual experience. In a case where you are married to a woman where the man's penis size and the woman's vaginal size is not a perfect match, then such couple would experience a little setback in the different sexual positions they can try out. So, thanks to Kama Sutra, we can make the right choice regarding the penis and vaginal sizes to enjoy a full sensual experience.

**3. Kama Sutra also emphasizes on living a healthy life and well-balanced one**

Kama Sutra is also a book that talks about tips on how to live a healthy life. The Kama Sutra encourages that a man and a woman should embrace cleanliness which would, in turn, boost their health. A man, for instance, should shave his beard on a regular basis, and take his bath and eat healthily, and the same applies to a woman too. She should bread her hair and shave as well. Couples could also try mutual grooming.

*4.Kama Sutra talks about enticing and approaching women*

The Kama Sutra also talks about interesting tips a man can use to entice and approaching a woman. This tip helps men to know how to touch and caress a woman in other to express their desire when they want to have sex. When a man knows these various tips and how to use them, he will find it easier to get his message over to the woman. The tips of how to entice and approach a woman further move on to touching and embracing.

*5.Kama Sutra talks about eight different types of embrace*

There are different types of embrace from the Kama Sutra. It further tells us that there are up to eight different types of embrace which can be used for different purposes. Because of Kama Sutra teaching, we now know how to apply the various types of embrace. And applying the right type of embrace at the right moment would set the right mood in motion. So, rather than keeping all your emotions inside, you can now use the various teaching from Kama Sutra about embrace to seduce and lure your lover into that perfect love zone.

*6.Kama Sutra teaches about kissing*

There are different forms of kissing too. Kama Sutra also teaches that a woman should feel too shy about a kiss. We all know that a man in most cases is the ones that initiate the kiss, but a woman should not feel shy to be the one to start the kiss first. There are also different types of kiss that partners can use to deeply connect with each other at particular points in your relationship. Like a type of kissing couples can engage in when walking on a lonely street. There are also different types of kiss that lovers can engage in when they want to make love.

*7.Kama Sutra is divided into a set of 64 acts*

Contrary to the belief that the Kama Sutra doesn't have a list of sex positions howbeit lovemaking that includes penetration is divided into 64 acts. This act explains the different ways couples can have sex to enjoy the maximum pleasure from sex. To have the best sex, you have to combine it with stimulating desire, and engaging in an embrace, caressing, kissing, biting, slapping, moans, oral sex, and everything in-between.

*8.Kama Sutra recommends that your scratch your partner*

There are different types of scratch you can have with your partner. With this knowledge Kama Sutra provides us, we can add a twist to lovemaking without loved ones. Moreover, leaving scratch marks on your lover's body can help keep the fire burning for each other even when your lover is not close to you.

*9.Kama Sutra recommends that your woman lover should reach orgasm first*

When making love with our loved once, Kama Sutra suggests that the woman should be the first to have an orgasm. This point is valid because of the extreme exhaustion a man feels after having an orgasm, whereby he wouldn't be able to proceed with sex at least not immediately. So, in other to have great sex, the woman should be the first to have an orgasm before the man allows himself to have an orgasm.

*10.Kama Sutra also talks about a woman's sex as being more than just sex penetrations*

In Kama Sutra, there is more to sex than penetration for a woman. To a woman, the whole act is sensual, but to a man reaches orgasm at the end of the intercourse. Most men think that making a woman have an orgasm is their ultimate act, but a woman needs both sexual and physiological pleasure to be able to satisfy her urge. Thanks to Kama Sutra, many men who were getting this concept wrong have been able to make adjustments.

# Chapter 11: How to Last Longer

Individuals who truly care for their partner want to extend the closeness and passion only lovemaking can bring. These people love to stay close to their partner (both physically and emotionally). After completing a whole round of lovemaking, many couples like to talk about things that are important to their relationship.

One of the most important parts of a great sexual relationship is the ability to share what you like and dislike about your lovemaking sessions. If you can freely communicate these things with your partner, you'll have great opportunities of improving your passionate encounters. That means you can enhance the overall experience brought about by the union of your bodies.

However, after a few minutes (or hours) of meaningful conversations, you might want to make love to your partner again. In this situation, the woman often needs to masturbate her partner to get his "member" erect again.

Important Note: If the couple doesn't want to have sex again, but the female isn't satisfied yet, the best thing a man can do is masturbate his lover until she reaches orgasm.

## How to Rekindle the Sexual Excitement

- The following techniques can help you prepare your partner for another round of lovemaking:
- The woman must use one of her hands to fondle the testicles of her partner. Her other hand, meanwhile, should slide up and down the penis.
- Once the penis is starting to become erect, the woman must brush it using her palm. She should make light, circular strokes using the palm of her hand.

## Helping a Woman to Achieve Orgasm

If your lover hasn't reached a climax during sex, or if she likes to have another orgasm but you are still not ready for a new round, you may stimulate her clit using your hands and fingers.

## How to Sustain the Harmony

In general, couples don't like to throw away the warmth of passionate lovemaking by simply falling asleep, or by doing things that are mentally or physically demanding. Some lovers want to lie on the bed and feel each other's presence, while others like to perform a gentle (but not sensual) massage.

If the couple wants to get up from the bed, they can sustain the romantic and harmonious mood by listening to music, eating together, or walking leisurely.

**What You Can Do After**

The Kama Sutra offers excellent techniques that can help extend the post-sex intimacy between the man and the woman. Some of these techniques are:

- After making love to each other, the couple should clean themselves separately. Once this is done, the couple must sit together–the man will apply some lotion on the woman's body.
- The man must embrace his partner and tell her how he appreciates her. Then, he should offer her some water to drink.
- The couple may eat fruits, sweetmeats, or anything they like. Also, they may drink soup, gruel, or fresh juice.

# Chapter 12: Exercises to increase male orgasmic control

The first of these is a very simple technique that doesn't require a great deal of explanation, or much imagination to understand. To illustrate, imagine (if you're a male reader) that you're at the proctologist's office. As you assume the position, you hear the familiar, rubberized "snap" behind you, as the good doctor dons his surgical gloves. You know his next move is to insert his finger in a place you'd rather he didn't.

Most male readers will have experienced a pronounced contraction of their anal sphincters as they read the foregoing account. This is a natural, defensive response at the prospect of a foreign object (the proctologist's probing finger), being inserted in the anus. But if you practice this movement regularly, consciously and gradually increase the duration of anal contractions as you grow stronger, you will soon be able to control ejaculation during intercourse. The contraction of the anal sphincter serves the purpose of preventing orgasm from occurring before you want it to. This is an easy method, but one that takes a little time, patience and practice. Starting with 30 repetitions, you'll soon find that the contraction of these muscles is easy and takes very little effort on your part.

Another technique involves the small area between the male testicles and the anus. This area, when pressed, inhibits the ability of sperm to flow to the shaft of the lingam and then, be ejaculated. Placing a finger on this spot and applying pressure at the right moment will stop ejaculation from occurring.

Finally, squeezing the shaft of the yoni, when the male senses ejaculation is imminent, can serve to stop climax from occurring. Firmly gripping and then squeezing the shaft works as a way of distracting the mind from the impending orgasm, allowing the man to continue with sex by delaying it.

Sexual continence is a much more achievable goal for women. Generally speaking, orgasm is more of a long term project for women and thus, not the great issue it is for men. The male climax can arrive at inopportune moments; moments at the woman partner is far from happy with her experience. This is an impediment to arriving at the divine state of sexual union that eludes so many of us.

Despite the more time-consuming nature of female orgasm, it's also advisable that women use the breathing exercises outlined in this section. Delaying their own orgasms can lead to the type of cosmic orgasm I've described elsewhere in this book. Learning to breathe slowly and intentionally and live in the sexual moment is not just for men. It's for women, too. You're both in this together and a little solidarity, as the male partner seeks to delay his orgasm, can be a strong binding agent and yet another way to increase the sexual bond between you.

## Kegels – strengthening the Yoni

Many women today practice Kegel exercises. These can serve to help women regain the yoni's natural elasticity, following childbirth, as well as restore their ability to retain urine for long periods of time (which can be effected by childbirth, also). For those of you reading though, Kegel exercises are a way to strengthen the muscles of the yoni, in order to be able to use them as a way to increase both your pleasure and that of your partner.

The muscles engaged when using Kegel exercises are those located in the pelvic floor. If readers are unsure as to where they are and how to "flex" them, they can find them by stopping the flow of urine the next time they visit the washroom. The muscles that stop the flow are those we're looking for. Women readers can practice doing this several times, until they can engage these muscles when they're not urinating. Also, Kegel exercises shouldn't be used to stop the flow of urine as a habit. This can lead to the bladder getting the message that it should retain some of the urine it needs to eliminate and can result in bladder infections, which most will agree are very unpleasant.

Kegel exercises, practiced as a series of contractions and releases can be started by holding the engagement of these pelvic floor muscles for a count of five. A good place to start is with a set of ten of these. Once readers feel they've mastered this stage of development, they can move on to ten sets of ten count contractions, resting for ten seconds between each. Making a habit of doing these exercises every day, will result in readers having the ability to amaze their partners with their superior muscle control. Male partners may be screaming for mercy, once their women have Kegeled their way to stronger yonis!

## Exercise for better sex

Some will not much care to hear this, but it needs to be said. Physical fitness makes sex a lot more fun. Especially if you're planning on practicing sexual continence for prolonged love making, the last thing you want is to get tuckered out before you've gotten anywhere near that sexual ecstasy you're hoping for.

Of particular importance is cardiovascular health. We've all heard stories of people who've suffered cardiac events in the throes of passion. If you're concerned that might end up being you, then it's time to take the bull by the horns and treat your heart to more of what it needs – exercise. All exertion will become easier for you and your sexual encounters will be effortless, when you're not concerned that your heart may not be meeting the challenge.

Walking regularly is a pleasant and healthy way to get more exercise and it's also an enjoyable activity you can do with the god or goddess in your life, as you plan your new life of sexual connection and fulfillment. You don't have to run a marathon. You don't have to scale Everest. You just need to feel your best, because part of being the best possible version of yourself is your wellness. You and your partner will thank me later, even if the thought of exercise leaves you cold now.

Another extremely effective form of exercise is planking (which comes to us from the world yoga, discussed below). While some of you may believe this is too challenging, planking is achievable for people of almost every fitness level. It is a silver bullet that engages a broad array of the body's muscle groups. Start by holding the plank for ten seconds, adding additional time as you're able. Soon you'll find that your posture and muscle tone have improved dramatically, as you're able to hold the plank for longer periods of time. There is also a strong meditative aspect to the plank, when held for longer duration. This type of focus will serve you well, as you seek the divine in your sex life, together.

If you're not sure how to properly execute a plank, be sure to explore online resources, or consult with a fitness professional in your area. Planking, in only a few minutes every day, can make you much stronger and more physically ready to enter into a world of erotic delight with your partner.

## Yoga

Yoga is a natural ally of those who are undertaking the spiritualization of their sexuality. Yoga can help prepare your bodies for the sexual journey you're embarking on by attuning it to the project.

Yoga incorporates its own type of breath control, which is called "pranayama". This type of breathing is responsible for releasing oxytocin into the bloodstream, which enhances the sex drive (see further on in this section for more on pranayama). An added benefit is an improved flow of blood to your genitals, which adds to the effect of the breathing techniques involve. Yoga has also been proven to help men achieve erections of longer duration and increased testosterone production. Following are some simple poses to begin with, which are specifically geared to improving stamina and strength for more effortless sex. Perhaps you'll find you enjoy yoga and want to go further with your practice. In that case, there's no shortage of yoga studios just about anywhere the world you can think of, as yoga has become the aerobics of the 21st Century.

## The Chair

This pose is particularly useful for women, as it engages the muscles of the pelvic floor in the same way the Kegel exercises do (see above in this section). The practice of this pose, then, is a good compliment to women using the Kegel to strengthen their yonis' ability to grip the male lingam.

As you perform this pose, pretend you're about to sit in a chair. Stand with your feet together and touching. Now, bend your knees as you would to become seated in a chair, bent slightly forward from the waist. Raise your arms over your head, relaxed, but elongated. Now consciously elongate the lowest part of your spine (tailbone/coccyx). By engaging the muscles in your pelvic floor, this part of your spine will be pulled back and straightened, aligning your upper body. Make sure to engage your abdomen and back muscles. Hold for as long as you're comfortable with. As you become stronger, you'll be able to hold this and other poses longer.

**The Squat**

This pose is exactly what it sounds like. You will perform a deep squat. Beneficial for the muscles of your inner thighs, the squat also engages the pelvis and serves to promote the health of all the joints in this region of the body. Your abdominal muscles are also engaged. It's believed by some that your spleen and reproductive system are stimulated by this pose, also.

With your feet apart at just a little beyond the width of your hips, your toes should be turned out. Now bring the palms of your hands together and place them directly in front of you, centered over the chest area. Now lower yourself toward the floor. Get as low as you can, comfortably, without straining yourself. Keeping your spine long and engaging your abdominal muscles will yield the greatest benefit of this pose. If you're able and wish to stretch your inner thighs, you can use your elbows to push your knees out further.

The squat can also be performed with the feet wide apart (toes still pointed out). This is probably the more realistic option for beginners, as it's somewhat less demanding. In this variation, lower yourself to the level of your knees, with your arms up and bent at the elbow, palms facing forward.

**The Cobra**

This well-known yoga pose is an excellent stretch for the abdominal muscles and for the associated muscle group that extends into the genital region and the pelvis. This is an excellent pose couples can engage in immediately before a session of prolonged sex.

Lying on your stomach with your legs together, push yourself up with your palms flat to support the weight of your upper body. Make sure to engage your abdominal muscles when you do this, in order to protect your back. If you're a beginner, keep the neck long and the head facing forward, as you imagine pressing your pelvis into the floor. Once you've become accustomed to this pose, you can pull your head back to look up, taking great care not to strain your neck and remembering to hold your shoulders down (don't let them drift up to your ears, as this aspect of the pose strengthens the arms, shoulders and upper back).

If you find this classical version of the cobra too difficult, you can raise yourself on your elbows, with your forearms extended in front of you. This will not achieve the deep stretch of the classic, but it's safer if it's been a while since you engaged in any type of deep stretching activity. Safety first! It's difficult to engage in prolonged lovemaking when your neck is out!

**Pranayama breathing**

In Sanskrit, "prana" means "life force". By learning to breathe in a way that allows the life force to flow through you unobstructed, you are releasing its power.

A fitting introduction to this type of breathing is the "Challenger" (known in Sanskrit as "ujjayi pranayama", which means "hissing breath"). Let's review how it's accomplished, step by step.

This style of pranayama produces a gentle hiss, as the breath is drawn in and out, over the posterior section of the throat. This may sound difficult, but if you practice it mindfully and intentionally, you'll learn how to do it.

Seat yourself in the lotus position (or modified lotus, if you find the classic version uncomfortable). You can also seat yourself in a chair, with your back straight and your shoulders relaxed. Both feet should be flat on the floor, if seated. Your hands may be placed in your lap, the right hand over the left, palms up and thumbs touching.

Draw your breath in through your nose, exhaling through your open mouth. As you breathe in and out, consciously seek to draw your breath across the back of your throat. For the exhale, accompany it with a protracted "ha". After repeating your exhalation and inhalation a few times, close your mouth. You're now going to do the same, using your nose for both inhalations and exhalations.

As you inhale and exhale, visualize your breath flowing across the back of the throat. As you do this, you should be hearing a gentle hissing (for which this type of pranayama is named). This is known as the "unspoken mantra" and its benefits are threefold. Your breathing will become slower. The sound also helps your mind to focus on your breathing and prevent it from adhering to stray thoughts that may distract you. As you monitor the hissing sound, ensuring that it maintains the same quality from beginning to end of your breaths, your flow is naturally rendered more smooth.

Practicing the challenger style of breathing can begin with a five to eight-minute session, which you may gradually increase to ten and eventually, fifteen minutes. When you've completed your breathing practice, you should revert to breathing as you normally do, still either in the lotus, or seated, for several minutes. Following this, lay down for a little while to return to your normal frame of mind and to absorb what you're feeling as the result of your breathing practice.

With time and dedicated practice, you'll find that the benefits of ujjayi pranayama include quieting your mind, which allows increased focus in every area of life and, of course, in your sexual practice. When both partners practice breathing in this way together, the mutual benefits will soon become apparent in your lovemaking. Synchronizing your breath to one another and using some of the techniques found in this chapter will prove enormously helpful for strengthening your connection with each other and supporting extended lovemaking – especially when sexual continence is being practiced.

# Chapter 13: How to Apply Everything you've Learnt about Kama Sutra

When you can successfully apply everything, you have learned from this book, you would experience a bit change in your sexual life. Now, if you are feeling a bit confused on how to apply Kama Sutra, don't worry I've got you covered. I've put together five easy to learn a step-by-step process you can follow to apply Kama Sutra to your love life successfully.

**1. Approach your lover**

The first and most important thing you need to do is first to make an approach. If you do not make a harmless approach, you would never know what your partner loves, and what they don't. There are different ways you can approach your lover about the whole idea of the Kama Sutra. Many people often prefer to just come out clean with the whole idea of the Kama Sutra, which normally works for them. They often come back with a smile on their face that simply talking with their partner was all they needed.

However, it isn't everyone that is endowed with this gift. So, if you know deep down your lover would have second thoughts about the Kama Sutra, don't bother approaching her with a conversation of the Kama Sutra, rather show it to her. Make her feel a difference in you, more like a new you.

## 2. Make an Attempt

Next step you are to take after deciding what approach you want to use to lure your partner into Kama Sutra, is to make an attempt. Now, this step is very crucial as you wouldn't want to rush things a little too much. So, start with the basics. Don't attempt with her with difficult sex positions; in fact, try to avoid the sex positions when you start. Keep your attempts to foreplay and kissing.

You don't want to speak your lover or make them feel disgusted by the Kama Sutra because they are not used to it. And you know what they say about the first impression, it last longer. So, make sure you give your lover a really memorable first impression. Make her feel those sensations, touch her at those sensitive points we talked about the erogenous zones. Play around with her, make her laugh, make her feel something so sensual that she'd have to close her eyes and open her mouth because she can't hold it in altogether.

## 3. Seduce

When you're making the right attempt, and it seems to be working, that is just perfect because what you're going to do next is to go for the seduction part. This could be the part where you add a little massage to the mix. Try massaging her with oil, or better still dry but make it a full naked both massage. Then as you massage her, occasionally go towards her buttocks, go towards her vaginal area, and stimulate the clitoris from time to time. And don't forget also to rub and massage the breast as well.

For the man, be sure to massage his penis and around his balls, a blow job too would go a long way in causing arousal. Seduction should be very sensual and filled with so much emotion. If you want to do it right, make sure the environment is conducive. We've spoken about making the environment perfect, so be sure to employ it the right way. Make the room warm when it is cold outside, or cold wand well aerated when it is warm outside.

## 4. Go for any of the sex positions you've learned

When you have finally groomed your lover to the extent that all they can think about is sex with you, then you're halfway there. At this point, this is when you are going to apply the best sex position you've learned. Also, don't start with something too difficult. Go for something very simple, something very pleasurable, and something that is more of pleasure than of a sex position itself.

As soon as you go for in penetration, be sure to take things slowly at first. Don't also forget to stimulate other parts of her body as you continue to make love to her. Then feel free to change sex position from time to time as you progress in love.

## 5. Try an after sex fun

Last but not least, after sex, you can engage in a conversation with your lover. Ask him or her what they like about sex, so you can know where to shift and make an adjustment. With time, you'd only get better and making romantic hot crazy sex with your lover.

# Conclusion

Comfort can be a misleading term regarding relationships and sex. Stepping out of your comfort zone to try new things will only make you more comfortable than you were before, in the future. It is a difficult concept to grasp, but it is so important to change things up and keep them changing in order to avoid repetition and boredom. No one wants to describe their love and sex life as boring; it is up to you and only you to make sure that does not happen. Sexual satisfaction can be done with or without the addition of toys, other individuals, and different geographic locations, but sexual exploration cannot. As a human being, you can decide if sexual adventure is what you are looking for or it sexual ritualism is something you are looking into. Next time you and your loved one take to bed, take a look at this book and see if there are any positions in which you might be interested in trying or experimenting with. Regardless of your relationship or sexual status as of this moment, this book was intended to be educational for the purpose of sexual exploration and sexual adventurism. Happy lovemaking!

www.ingramcontent.com/pod-product-compliance
Lightning Source LLC
Chambersburg PA
CBHW070904080526
44589CB00013B/1179